NI

Future Tense, or... Tense Future

For Pam—
Good luck as
you ride the waves
of change. Venner
5-13-98

Venner M. Farley Ed.D., R.N.

ISBN 1-888315-00-8

Printed in the United States of America

DEDICATION

To my colleagues in nursing who see the wisdom in willingly thinking and acting in different ways.

ACKNOWLEDGMENTS

As always to Dee whose confidence keeps me going; and to Nell Magnera who has turned my tapes into chapters of a book. Thanks to Bob Anderson at KNI for his intelligent counsel; and to Roy Anderson who prepared the final design of the book.

Published by:

Innovative Nursing Consultants (INC)
6512 E. Kings Crown Road
Orange, Ca. 92669
(714) 744-2814

About The Author

VENNER M. FARLEY, Ed.D., R.N. Dr. Farley is a nationally known expert in the field of nursing education, nursing management and shared governance. Known for her wit and wisdom, Dr. Farley is able to analyze current trends in nursing and offer meaningful strategies for survival.

Dr. Farley was Dean of Health Professions at Golden West College, in Huntington Beach, California. Prior to that, she had a long history of academic involvement. She is widely respected and speaks to nurses across the nation on topics such as empowerment, professionalism and strategic planning. The author of numerous articles including "Clinical Teaching: A Shared Adventure" and "Yesterday is a Dream Tomorrow is a Vision - Today is a Beginning." In 1995, Dr. Farley published the book Nurses Pulling Together to Make a Difference.

She earned her doctorate at the University of Southern California in higher education and administration. She is a member of the board of directors of Long Beach Memorial Medical Center in Long Beach, California and she chairs the Medical Affairs Committee for the board of directors of that institution. She is an elected governor-at-large of the National league for Nursing; and she is president and principal consultant of Innovative Nursing Consultants, in Orange, California.

NURSES: FUTURE TENSE OR TENSE FUTURE

Chapters

Preface

We are living on the edge of a new millennium and it is very painful...for our nation, for our world...and for our profession. Healthcare is re-inventing itself and this requires thinking and acting differently for all concerned: providers and consumers, to say nothing of employers and insurers.

Additionally, we are living in a time of enormous denial of all of the change that has already occurred; and we are uncomfortable with the realities that are becoming known to us. One example of a new reality in a world of discontinuous change is that of a time and a world without well defined and stable jobs.

The job-shifting of the late 20th Century is ruthless and scary for all our citizens; and this time physicians and nurses are very much a part of the concomitant chaos. Nurses have never before faced a time when their jobs are subject to re-definition, de-layering, re-structuring and market contingencies.

> America has entered the age of the contingent or temporary worker, of the consultant and subcontractor, of the just-in-time work force -fluid, flexible, disposable. This is the future. Its message is this: You are on your own. For good (sometimes) and ill (often). The workers of the future will constantly have to sell their skills, invent new relationships with employers who must, themselves, change and adapt constantly in order to survive in a ruthless global market.

Lance Morrow, "The Temping of America," Time, March 29, 1993

Nurses are being challenged by these changes as never before. The work of nurses and the work of nursing is in transition

because of societal mandates which are also inherent in the transitions needed to reform our healthcare system. It is imperative that nurses adopt new strategies in accepting the challenges presented to our profession. We must be fast, focused, fit, and flexible as we prepare to evolve (yes! evolve) nursing into the 21st Century healthcare market; and we must answer these questions:

1. What will the future healthcare system look like?
2. What skills will nurses need to survive in it?
3. How can you, the nurse, be in charge of your career when your employing agency is evaporating?
4. How do we forget what we have always done in nursing before it suffocates us?
5. How do we create the 21st Century professional nurse who answers this question: What is the essential healthcare service which customers need - and only RNs are providing?

The crux of nursing's transformation lies in having the courage to ask of ourselves: future tense...or tense future??? The answer lies within the nursing profession itself.

LORD, ARE YOU TRYING TO TELL ME SOMETHING?

FOR

FAILURE DOES NOT MEAN I'M A FAILURE;
IT DOES MEAN I HAVE NOT YET SUCCEEDED.
FAILURE DOES NOT MEAN I HAVE ACCOPLISHED NOTHING;
IT DOES MEAN I HAVE LEARNED SOMETHING.
FAILURE DOES NOT MEAN I HAVE BEEN A FOOL;
IT DOES MEAN I HAD ENOUGH FAITH TO EXPERIMENT.
FAILURE DOES NOT MEAN I'VE BEEN DISGRACED;
IT DOES MEAN I DARED TO TRY.
FAILURE DOES NOT MEAN I DON'T HAVE IT;
IT DOES MEAN I HAVE TO DO SOMETHING IN A DIFFERENT WAY.
FAILURE DOES NOT MEAN THAT I AM INFERIOR;
IT DOES MEAN THAT I AM NOT PERFECT.
FAILURE DOES NOT MEAN THAT I HAVE WASTED MY LIFE;
IT DOES MEAN THAT I HAVE AN EXCUSE TO START OVER.
FAILURE DOES NOT MEAN THAT I SHOULD GIVE UP;
IT DOES MEAN THAT I MUST TRY HARDER.
FAILURE DOES NOT MEAN THAT I WILL NEVER MAKE IT;
IT DOES MEAN THAT I NEED MORE PATIENCE.
FAILURE DOES NOT MEAN YOU HAVE ABANDONED ME;
IT DOES MEAN YOU HAVE A BETTER IDEA.

AMEN

ANONYMOUS

CHAPTER 1

THE TANGLED WEB OF CAPITATION AND MANAGED CARE

Einstein: *"How do I work...I grope."*

The future for healthcare delivery in the USA lies in a capitated, managed care environment called an integrated healthcare delivery system. The effects of this development on nursing cannot be oversold and nurses need to understand what each of these terms means.

Managed Care - A system of discounted healthcare in which the care of customers is "managed" by physicians and hospitals to produce the desired outcome for a discounted fee contracted via insurance companies, e.g., a preferred provider organization (PPO).

Capitation - In this evolving system, the fee for managing the healthcare of participants is paid "up front" at a "per member/per month" rate. The providers must then "manage" the customers' healthcare so as to obtain quality outcomes, while still achieving a profit at the end of the month. The best examples of this are the health maintenance organizations (HMO) emerging all over the country.

Integrated Delivery Systems - These are full service systems providing care to customers via a seamless continuum of options managed by primary care providers (internists, family practice physicians, nurse practitioners, etc.). This seamless continuum of care has within it a range of services from clinics and physicians' offices to satellite centers to home care agencies to surgi-centers to community hospitals to tertiary medical centers. It is well recognized that the use of hospital care will be greatly minimized in order to control the cost of health care and disease prevention.

Healthcare reform is evolving so rapidly that it is difficult and very risky to predict exactly what the system will be in 5-10 years. However, there are specific "eternal truths" which have emerged which will be the foundations on which reform must be based:

1. The healthcare provider must be able to demonstrate high quality healthcare outcomes.
2. Customers must be satisfied (people who receive care and the employers who pay for it, as well as the contractors/ insurance companies who formulate the contract between employers and providers).
3. The provider must be able to deliver #1 and #2 at a cost that is 15-25% below current market costs (Long Beach Memorial Medical Center: "Strategic Plan for Care Lines," 1995).

Recognizing that the implications of these revolutionary changes are gigantic for hospitals and physicians is relatively easy for nurses. Accepting that such changes are having an enormous impact on the practice of nursing is much more difficult. These profound changes on the triad of hospitals, physicians, and nurses are all related to the economics of healthcare delivery. Since the rising costs have thus far been intractable, we must be clear sighted enough to see that the development of a system that rationally manages the cost of healthcare and the cost of disease care is and will remain the focal point of healthcare reform in this country.

This quotation is from a Modern Healthcare editorial, June 12, 1995:

> Managing disease will require improving out-comes data, revamping the way physicians and nurses operate, cutting inpatient admissions, shortening hospital stays, and eliminating unnecessary diagnostic tests and medical procedures. No quick or easy solutions here. But only fundamental systemic change holds the promise of truly reforming medical care delivery and, in the end, reducing costs.

Nurses must accept the fact that as hospitals re-define themselves, and physicians re-define the practice of medicine, so must we, as nurses, re-define our practice. If 85% of healthcare will be delivered OUTSIDE of hospitals, the practice of nursing will also be re-deployed, re-structured, re-designed to fit the new system. The key question for nurses is whether or not we will do it ourselves, or, once again, will we allow it to be done unto us?

This tangled web of healthcare reform will go on and on for many years. Mistakes will be made...and rectified. Experiments will be tried...and many will fail. Count on what Winston Churchill said in World War II: "Americans can be counted on to do the right thing - once they have tried everything else."

So these transitions of healthcare reform are scary and painful for all those involved: customers and providers (hospitals, physicians, nurses, etc.). This turbulent environment is chaotic. And only through the chaos can the tangled web become transformed. Remember: The pain is inevitable; but suffering is your option.

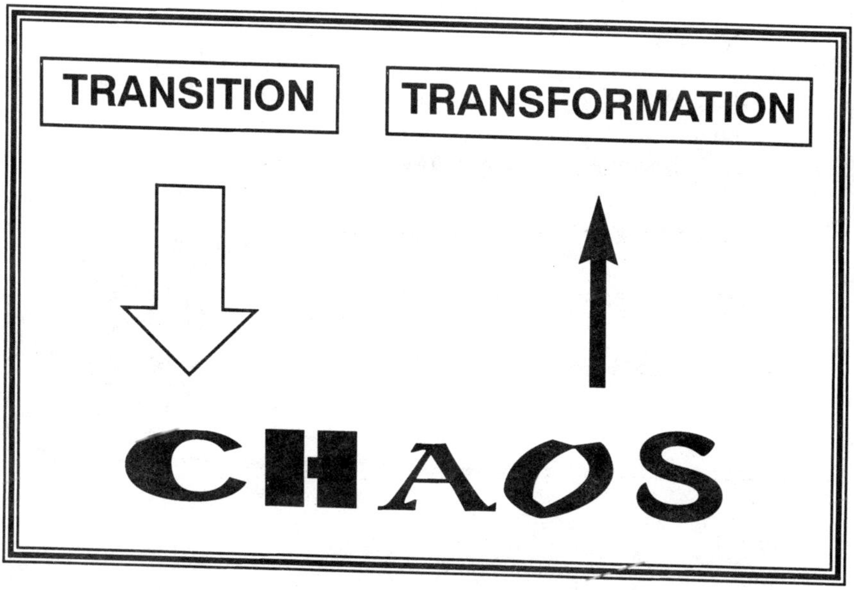

The future healthcare elements are relatively clear:

- Budget-managed, integrated delivery systems;
- Increased access to primary care;
- Primary care providers as gatekeepers;
- Measurable quality and service;
- Ambulatory orientation;
- Regional coverage;
- Major economic re-structuring.

FUTURE H.C. ELEMENTS

- BUDGET-MANAGED HEALTHCARE
- INC. ACCESS
- MEASURABLE QUALITY & SERVICE
- AMBULATORY ORIENTATION
- REGIONAL COVERAGE
- MAJOR ECONOMIC "RE-STRUCTURING"

Inherent in these elements is the recognition of fundamental changes in medical practice and the transition of hospitalization from a revenue producer (profit-maker) to a cost center.

KEY CHANGES

FROM	TO
Fee-For-S	Capitation
Specialty	Primary
Revenue Center	Cost Center
Fragments	Int. Entities
Local	Regional

The catalyzing events that are causing these changes in the delivery and reimbursement of healthcare are market driven, and that is what makes the prediction of constant change reasonable:

- Payor/insurer re-positioning;
- Small group reform demanded by employers;
- ncentives for medicaid and medicare customers contracting with HMOs;
- Continued government action to reform healthcare entitlements.

It is very likely that overall there will be fewer payors; and those which do survive and flourish will make quality and service i.e., customer satisfaction, a very high priority. Nurses, therefore, will be crucial to the delivery of value-added outcome achievement.

Outcomes

A way to measure values!

Value can be defined as outcome over (or divided by) cost. Nurses have enormous influence on customers discerning value in service; and on customer satisfaction with the quality of service received.

For example, the customer's evaluation of a satisfactory outcome is based on the customer's satisfaction with the outcome itself. This is based on how closely the outcome achieved matches up with the customer's own treatment goal.

FUTURE HEALTH SYSTEM

1. VERTICAL INTEGRATION
2. GEOGRAPHIC INTEGRATION
3. CAPITATION
4. LOW COST

Since nursing schools first opened in this country, nurses have been valued and respected because of their orientation toward "caring" in all of its parameters. The new roles for nurses will extend those domains by focusing on the registered nurse as "organizer and manager of managed care." Outcome achievement will be a primary domain of nurses in all places where healthcare is provided. This means an elaboration in the roles of nurse as teacher of customers and families in disease prevention, and health promotion. The desired outcomes must be achieved in time to both satisfy the customer and earn a profit for the providers within the integrated healthcare delivery system.

THE VIEWS FROM THE BED ON OUTCOMES

- Physical Function
- Social Function
- Energy
- Fatigue
- Pain

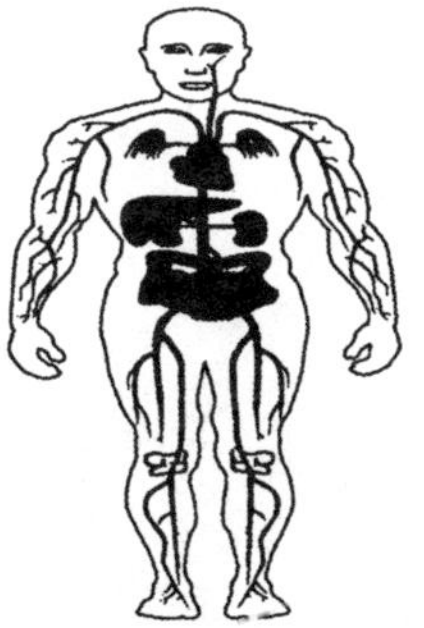

The question for nurses within this new framework is:

> What do we want nursing to look like in 5 years...and how are we going to get there?

In summary, the future healthcare system will be economically driven to provide the management of healthcare services that promote health, and prevent disease, offering a continuum of services that provide choices for venues of care along that continuum. But make no mistake, customer choice will be limited by capitated healthcare plans, and low cost will be the dominant factor in selection.

The pressures are building for change based on economic demands to alter the spiraling cost of healthcare; and the changes we see in the next 5-7 years will be startling and radical.

SUCCESS

SUCCESS IS NOT MEASURED BY HOW YOU DO

COMPARED TO HOW SOMEBODY ELSE DOES.

SUCCESS IS MEASURED BY HOW YOU DO

COMPARED TO WHAT YOU COULD HAVE DONE

WITH WHAT GOD GAVE YOU.

ANONYMOUS

CHAPTER 2

MAKING A DIFFERENCE: MAKING A PROFIT

If a house is divided against itself;
that house cannot stand.
St. Mark, 3:25

Leaders in nursing, some of whom used to be called managers, must recognize that nurses will rise to the challenges of healthcare reform and the concurrent reform of nursing when nurses accept these challenges as their very own. As the president of SAS has said: "An individual without information cannot take responsibility; an individual with information cannot help but take responsibility." So the key is shared information.

In the forthcoming capitated way of life in healthcare, nurses must understand that when healthcare providers, i.e., integrated delivery systems, accept capitated rates, they agree to provide whatever care is needed to a specified population for a fixed, monthly fee. When all goes well, that monthly fee will cover expenses and even yield a profit. Of course, there is a risk that the fee will not stretch far enough...and thus the fact that in capitation the risk is on the provider.

This is exactly the point at which nurses become a critical element. Nurses will rise to the challenge of managed/capitated care... when it is their challenge. There are two principles that will guide nursing leaders as they work to bring nurses into this equation:

1. The nurse doing the work must own the responsibility.
2. If you want nurses to act like it's their business...make it their business (Belasco, 1994).

M → **Maximize Employer Potential**

O → **Offer Opportunity For Growth**

T → **Trust Employees To Do Their Jobs**

I → **Involve Employees In Decisions**

V → **Value Employee Differences**

A → **Allow For Mistakes**

T → **Throw Away Threats & Punishments**

E → **Encourage Through Praise & Rewards**

Motivating the nurse at the practice level, coaching for self-motivation, and keeping the motivated nurse motivated is the essence of leadership for the 21st Century. It will be the way to make a profit in a capitated system because nursing for quality service at low cost is the key ingredient. It really does all come down to economics as the driving force in healthcare reform; and to nurses as the driving force in reducing risk for integrated delivery systems.

Nurse leaders and nurses at the practice level have begun to see that standing still is simply not an option, as the ground (the current healthcare system) is erupting all around us:

- Moving and changing in nursing and in nurses is essential behavior;
- Changing = learning & growing...not always without pain.

As leaders recognize that their requisite behaviors for leading (not managing) have changed, so nurses at the practice level must recognize that their practice now requires more in knowledge-based work. Nursing education at all levels, i.e., generic/basic preparation through graduate education, must move curricula quickly into meeting the new age demands on nurses.

NURSING ED. & SERVICE

Moves from labor intensive to knowledge-based work:

- **Assessment**
- **Analysis**
- **Planning**

SERVICE!!

Attempting to fathom these behaviors, which encompass thinking and acting so differently, requires dialog between nurses who lead and those who practice. If leaders want to know what is preventing nurses from great performance today...they will have to:

1. Ask nurses: "What is keeping you from great performance in your practice?"
2. Then, the leader must exert great effort to remove the obstacles identified (Belasco, 1994).

The "monitarization" of healthcare means different things to each of the participants. To the consumer of healthcare it means becoming aware of the providers' economic motives, and the possibility of conflicts of interest. It also means having a concern about quality and service and accuracy and truthfulness in healthcare delivery.

To providers in integrated delivery systems it means real worry about survival. Can we give quality care and service and make a profit? How can we ensure a profit - which really is essential for survival? Is there a quick and easy...and ethical way to survive? How much downsizing, de-layering and restructuring can a system take before it breaks down?
Physicians' concerns are just as tied up with quality, service, ethical issues, and profit-making as the other participants. And they are just as unprepared for changes as are nurses, because their education has not prepared them for collaboration, primary care practice, and the decision-making that healthcare economics demands in an integrated delivery system.

We even have a new vocabulary developing to articulate these concerns:

NEW WORDS:

- Assessment
- Analysis
- Planning
- Paradigm Shift
- Job Shift
- Privatization
- Catastrophyzing
- De-Jobbing
- Power Shift

ETC. ETC. ETC.

To assist consumers, physicians, and nurses in understanding the need for such profound changes in healthcare delivery, specific questions must be answered within the scope of each person's concern. When leaders have failed to answer those questions/ concerns failure has resulted. Re-engineering, re-structuring, de-layering fails when internal and external customers:

1. Lack adequate information.
2. Have not been given answers to the question, "Why?"
3. Have not been helped to see what is in these changes for them - what is the advantage to them, personally?

For nurses and physicians there are two additional factors for failure:

- Inadequate training, education and re-training and reeducation;
- No rewards or recognition for those who do make valuable contributions to the developing systemic changes.

An editorial in Modern Healthcare on May 15, 1995 stated that "A lot of snake oil has been sold in the name of TQM, CQI, downsizing, rightsizing, re-engineering and patient-focused care." That editorial went on to say, "...of half the companies that trimmed 10% of their staffs, only 61% reduced costs and only 34% achieved higher productivity," (Modern Healthcare, 5-15-95).

In his new book, one of the fathers of re-engineering, James Champy has written that, "Payoffs appear to have fallen short of their potential," (Champy, 1995).

Nurse leaders must pay heed. None of this means that experimentation should cease, on the contrary, new approaches must be tried. But nurse leaders must help build new practice guidelines for nurses like these:

- Become multi-skilled...a quick change artist in nursing practice;
- Commit fully to your work...nursing is full of new opportunities;

- Speed up...you have no choice;
- Accept ambiguity and uncertainty...it is our new reality;
- Stay in school...you must learn, learn, learn to survive in a knowledge-based practice;
- Be accountable for the outcomes of your practice...we will hold you to them;
- Nursing must be "value-added" or it cannot survive;
- The customer really is JOB #1...we are a service center;
- You must manage your own career...and your own morale...you are in charge;
- FIX IT...don't just point at it;
- Alter your expectations of work...everything is changing...we are moving, moving, moving.

(Pritchitt 1994)

So making a difference when the password itself is change is scary, treacherous, and difficult. Combining all of that with needing to make a profit in order to survive is even more scary, more treacherous...and, of course, essential. So resilience in managing change is crucial (Berger, 1995).

Resilience in Change Management:

- **Positive**
- **Focused**
- **Flexible**
- **Organized**
- **Proactive**

And remember as Tom Peters says (Peters, 1995) "it's really true... regarding change...we ain't seen nothing yet...you can count on it."

1990-2000 = 50 Years of change

2000-2005 = 50 Years of change

IN 15 Yrs – 100 Years of change

"Faith Popcorn"

The key to making a difference and making a profit in nursing is great leadership. Peters says that the essence of leadership is emotion, not administration (Peters, 1995). To create a philosophy of leadership, Peters asks leaders to:

1. Make a list of the things you hated as you climbed the ladder to success;
2. Make a list of the obverse of your first list;
3. That's your leadership philosophy (Peters, 1995).

That's a crucial exercise for formal and informal nursing leaders to undertake, if they are looking to survive and thrive in the 21st Century. Success will be judged not by being a good nurse, but by getting 1,000 other nurses excited about nursing in the 21st Century. The leaders' energy must be committed to the growth of other nurses...who also want to continue to make a difference in their practice, and understand the need to make a profit for the integrated healthcare delivery system.

RN's Please Note
Needed Work Attitudes
& Behaviors:

- **Adaptability**
- **Appreciation of Ambiguity**
- **Accomplishment**
- **Access Ability**
- **Accessibility**

Adapted From: Millennium, 1995

Healthy Spirit in Leadership

- **Be Sensitive**
- **Play to Strength**
- **Flow**
- **Improve**
- **Enjoy White Water Rafting**
- **Encourage Group Steering**

ARE YOU A WINNER?

THE WINNER IS ALWAYS PART OF THE ANSWER.
THE LOSER IS ALWAYS PART OF THE PROBLEM.

THE WINNER ALWAYS HAS A PROGRAM.
THE LOSER ALWAYS HAS AN EXCUSE.

THE WINNER SAYS LET ME DO IT.
THE LOSER SAYS THAT'S NOT MY JOB.

THE WINNER SEES AN ANSWER FOR EVERY PROBLEM.
THE LOSER SEES A PROBLEM FOR EVERY ANSWER.

THE WINNER SAYS IT MAY BE DIFFICULT, BUT IT IS POSSIBLE.
THE LOSER SAYS IT MAY BE POSSIBLE, BUT IT'S TOO DIFFICULT.

A WINNER LISTENS.
A LOSER WAITS UNTIL IT'S TIME TO TALK.

WHEN A WINNER MAKES A MISTAKE,S/HE SAYS I WAS WRONG.
WHEN A LOSER MAKES A MISTAKE, S/HE SAYS IT WASN'T <u>MY</u> FAULT.

A WINNER SAYS I'M GOOD, BUT NOT AS GOOD AS I WANT TO BE.
A LOSER SAYS I'M NOT AS BAD AS A LOT OF OTHER PEOPLE.

A WINNER FEELS RESPONSIBLE FOR MORE THAN THE JOB.
A LOSER SAYS, 'HEY, I ONLY WORK HERE."

AUTHOR UNKNOWN

CHAPTER 3

THE REVOLUTION IN NURSING'S WORK

Many will work temporary or part-time - sometimes because that's the way they want it, and sometimes because that's all t hat is available.

Charles Handy, *The Age of Unreason*

Job security is an oxymoron.

Tom Peters, *The Pursuit of WOW*

Einstein on his theory of insanity:
Doing the same thing, and expecting different results.

We are living in a time such as occurs only every 2-3 hundred years. A time of such change, that the past has not prepared us for the future (Toffler & Toffler, 1995; Drucker, 1994). A time when most of the people working in our society were prepared in... and for...an age which has passed. Drucker says we are living, right now, in an age of social transformation unlike anything ever before experienced.

JOB SECURITY ??

DOWNSIZING

DELAYERING

NO TIME
LESS MONEY
↑ DEMANDS

"...work and work force...are all...qualitatively and quantitatively different not only from what they were in the first years of this century, but also from what has existed at any other time in history; in their configurations, in their processes, in their problems, and in their structures," (Drucker, Atlantic Monthly, 1994).

The Tofflers and Drucker also agree that we are currently witnessing the death of the blue collar worker; and the rise of "knowledge" workers. Knowledge workers require continuous formal education; and a willingness to continually acquire more theoretical and analytical skill. These facts have tremendous implications for nurses because we must recognize that our future work will be vastly different from the work for which our education and training prepared us. In fact, to quote Drucker (1994) again: "...how well an individual, an organization, an industry, a country, does in acquiring and applying knowledge will become the key competitive factor."

So, nursing's future success as a profession will depend on the willingness of nurses to recognize and accept the changes inherent in both society's and our profession's transformation. We are, indeed and in fact, witnessing the demise of the practice of nursing and of nursing education as we have experienced it since its establishment in the 1870s.

NURSING'S BUSINESS IN THE 21ST CENTURY

- ★ **INTEGRITY**
- ★ **RESPECT**
- ★ **EMPOWERMENT**
- ★ **VISION**
- ★ **COMMUNICATIONS**
- ★ **SACRIFICE**
- ★ **BUDGETS**
- ★ **CONFLICT**
- ★ **HUMILITY**

TRUST

FLOURISHES!!

The paradigm has shifted for society, for medicine, for hospitals, and for nursing. The demands of the healthcare market today cannot be met by depending on yesterday's education and training.

Such a time creates great havoc and chaos for those who wish to stay grounded in yesterday. This is a painful time for all who yearn for "the good old days." The real question is who shall determine what replaces the good old days...who determines the future of nursing?

There are many nurses running scared, who see this future and these demands in a negative light - who persist in seeing this revolution as the glass half empty. They are failing to see the opportunities that inevitably accompany change. The danger is that if nurses do not accept the challenges of the new opportunities, others in the allied health field surely will.

Nurses are facing challenges that will require the very best we have in leadership, energy, ingenuity, commitment, creativity, and hard work. The "good old days" are gone for good - and that fact is not debatable. The USA is facing similar challenges in finding solutions to our nation's current economic, social and political problems. Nursing is not alone.

Is nursing...are nurses...going to give up at this critical juncture in our development by hanging on to the past, by demanding that we must be allowed to continue doing our work as we have always done it, by shouting that our paradigm has not shifted? Surely, not! We have always shown that we have the essential ingredients of energy, intelligence, creativity, passion, caring - to forge ahead and re-define nursing's practice in light of the demands of the social transformation of our nation.

HOSPITALS IN 2001: INTEGRATED DELIVERY SYSTEMS

- ★ OFFSITE ER & OR
- ★ AMBULATORY CARE
- ★ SUBACUTE SERVICES
- ★ ALTERNATIVE Rx
- ★ CASE MANAGEMENT
- ★ OUTCOME BENCHMARKING
- ★ WELLNESS
- ★ FITNESS
- ★ EDUCATION
- ★ TELECOMMUNICATIONS

NSG.'S GROWTH TOO!

Change is seldom easy, but it is not optional. It is happening - it has happened. Our only choice is to look for opportunity in a re-structured healthcare delivery system; and create the momentum that will enable us to embrace the ambiguity and uncertainty that inevitably accompanies this kind of transition, chaos, and transformation.

I see nursing's glass as full - full of potential, if we are willing to "pick ourselves up, dust ourselves off, and start all over again," (Ziggy Cartoons by Wilson, (1995). This revolution in nursing's work is our greatest opportunity and our greatest challenge. Our customer is counting on us to be able to deliver on our social contract for "caring".

Re-structuring and the rapid movement to managed care are creating a climate of unprecedented chaos. This has caused system wide errors due to the chaos, fear, and noise in the providers' environment. The chaos will continue, and so will the errors. All nurses, therefore, are obligated to take an active role in reframing and re-defining the work of nursing. Questions we must ask ourselves include these:

- What is nursing?
- Who do we as nurses want to be in a reformed healthcare delivery system?
- Who are our customers: implicit and explicit?
- Who are our competitors as healthcare providers?
- What do nurses do better than anyone else?
- What do nurses do that no one else does?
- What are the three most important elements in the business of nursing?

Leadership will make all the difference as the profession begins to answer these questions. The confident leader will seek to re-distribute power, will delegate broadly, and give up enormous amounts of control in order to be free to know the nursing staff and help them in defining new roles. Encouraging nurses at the practice level will be the great role of nurse leaders: active listening; asking questions; and applause!!

The nurses at the practice level, i.e., those who do the real work of nursing, who have that kind of support, will think and behave differently.

They will find themselves engaged in a forward movement such as nursing has not experienced before. As empowered nurses working in highly effective and efficient teams, they will:

- Understand the core issues of healthcare reform;
- Define nursing's role within these core issues;
- Recognize that all nurses must be leaders;
- Recognize that all nurses must be managers of managed care;
- Think and behave differently than at any other time in their professional lives;

- Be proactive in seeking involvement in resolving problems that affect nursing and nurses;
- "Speak up, talk straight, and question when needed." (Adapted from Matejka and Dunning, 1995)

The secret ingredient that leaders must seek is to build a nursing unit/department in which every nurse feels a particular sense of ownership, even though, in truth, they have none (Helgeson, 1995).

For nurses, re-structuring means change; and change means insecurity. In such a period of societal reform and healthcare upheaval, how do we help nurses control their own destiny and revolutionize the work of nursing? The answer lies in thinking and behaving differently along five specific parameters:

1. Face reality as it is;
2. Be open and honest with everyone;
3. Don't manage...lead;
4. Change before you have to;
5. Recognize that nursing and nurses must seek and maintain a competitive advantage.

QUALITY WITH A DIFFERENCE

Q Question everything

U Understand or seek to understand

A Attitude is altitude.

L Learning organizations are crucial

I Integrity is requisite

T Treasure the community as a work place

Y Yearn for success

"Denial is crippling American Business" (Shechtman, 1994)... and the same can be said for the nursing profession. Of course, we'd be comfortable keeping everything the same, of course working without a net is terrifying. Of course, denial is the strongest mental mechanism for coping. But excessive denial is maladaptive and prevents progress. Nurses today must be:

- Fit;
- Fast;
- Focused;
- Flexible.

Nurses must have a great capacity for change in order to accept the challenges of creating our future. The rewards will be substantial: autonomy and independence within a framework of collaboration and colleagueship.

PROFESSIONAL NURSING PRACTICE

1. DEAL WILLINGLY WITH MORE ISSUES
2. WHOLE-SYSTEMS THINKING
3. CORE ISSUES...RAPIDLY
4. LEARN FROM EXPERIENCE
5. APPLICATION OF KNOWLEDGE TO PRACTICE
6. INTEGRATE LEARNING CONTINUOUSLY
7. COST - EFFICIENT, SUPERIOR PRACTICE & PERFORMANCE

THE REVOLUTION IN NURSING WORK

UNSKILLED WORKER ⟶ KNOWLEDGE WORK

REPETITIVE ⟶ INNOVATE & CHANGE

INDIVIDUAL WORK ⟶ SELF-MANAGED TEAMS

SINGLE SKILLED ⟶ MULTI-SKILLED

POWER BOSS ⟶ POWER COLLEAGUE

COMMUNICATE ⟶ TOP

COMMUNICATE ⟶ PEERS

Willful ignorance will be our greatest barrier to creating this future. Bear in mind these wise words from The Web of Inclusion by Sally Helgeson (1995):
Nothing in a living system can be regarded separately from the eventual consequences it creates for the larger environment. As Erich Jantsch points out in The Self-Organizing Universe, "In life, the issue is not control but dynamic connectedness."

LOOK AHEAD

VISION ASSURES HOPE FOR TOMORROW,

LAUGH

MERRIMENT PRODUCES SUNSHINE FOR THE SOUL,

LOVE

CARING IS A GIFT FOR ALL SEASONS,

LEARN

KNOWLEDGE FUELS THE FIRES OF GROWTH AND FREEDOM,

LIFT UP

A POSITIVE SPIRIT BUFFERS THE STORMS OF LIFE,

LET GO

FREEDOM FROM FEAR IS THE PASSPORT TO PEACE.

AUTHOR UNKNOWN

CHAPTER 4

NURSES: OUR WORK IS THINKING

The education and skills of the workforce will end up being the ultimate competitive weapon.
Lester Thurow

As nursing practice becomes outcome based, instead of task based, nurses must recognize the range of their cognitive abilities and fortify them purposefully.

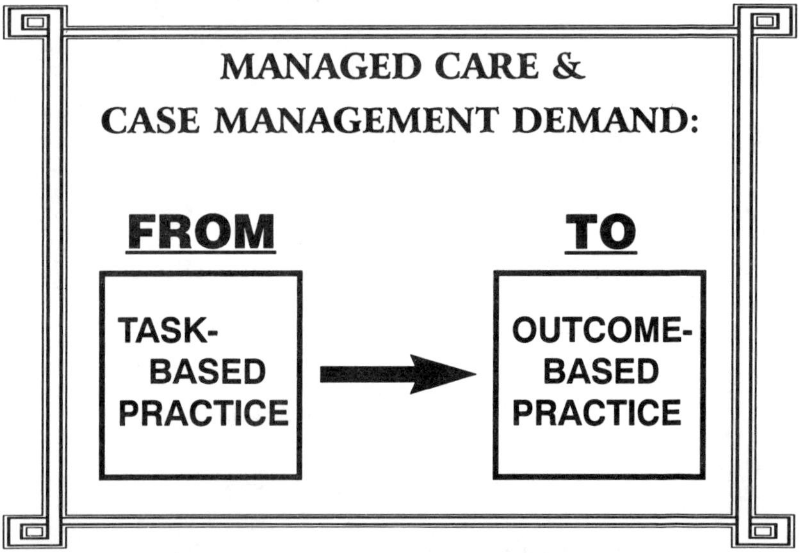

Thinking is a skill, an intellectual skill, and therefore it can be learned, practiced, and developed. Cognition has always been the foundation of excellent nursing practice, now it is time to articulate that fact, and actively promote it as the essence of our work.

The constant conversation about critical thinking in nursing education curricula over the last few years, is timely. Nurses always thought critically (more or less), but they probably did not know where the skill came from, or how it happened to be in their repertoire...probably serendipity or osmosis.

The nurse at the practice level needs to understand what thinking is, and that it must be purposeful in our assessment, analysis, and planning to achieve specific outcomes for our customers. For if intelligence is potential, then thinking is its' engine. DeBono puts it this way: "Thinking is the operating skill through which intelligence acts upon experience," (DeBono, 1994). He goes on to say:

> ...highly intelligent people need to improve their thinking skills in order to make full use of that high intelligence. Much of the potential of high intelligence is otherwise wasted, (DeBono, 1994).

AND

> So those who do not consider themselves highly intelligent can improve their performance by improving their thinking skill, (DeBono, 1994).

These facts are directly applicable to nurses and the practice of nursing. As nursing becomes a knowledge based profession, the future will belong to those who emphasize the intellectual components of nursing in their practice.

Drucker speaks of this as "a habit of continuous learning," (1994). In discussing the rise of the knowledge worker in the social transformation of our nation, which is occurring at this very moment, Drucker goes on to say:

> ...the great majority of the new job qualifications the industrial worker does not possess and is poorly equipped to acquire. They require a good deal of formal education and ability to acquire and to apply theoretical and analytical knowledge, (Drucker, 1994).

Although that message of Drucker's is not <u>directly</u> transferrable to nursing (we are <u>not</u> industrial workers), his point must be taken: nurses must move to a new appreciation of their thinking capacities, and continuously hone them to support their considerable psychomotor skills.

> Increasingly, an educated person will be somebody who has learned how to learn, and who continues learning, especially by formal education, throughout his or her lifetime, (Drucker, 1994).

Purposeful thinking in nursing enables nurses to:

- Be flexible in adapting to a changing healthcare environment;
- focus on decision making and judgement-calling in outcome based practice;
- maintain a continuous track for learning in our personal and professional lives.

We cannot settle for less.

Alfaro (1995) produced this definition of critical thinking and its application to nursing practice:

> Unlike the "mindless" thinking we do when going about our daily routines, critical thinking is purposeful, goal-directed thinking that aims to make judgments based on evidence (fact), rather than conjecture (guesswork). Based on principles of science and the scientific method (e.g., maintaining a questioning attitude, following an organized approach to discovery, and making sure information is reliable) critical thinking requires the developing strategies that maximize human potential (e.g., tapping on individual strengths) and compensate for problems caused by human nature (e.g., the powerful influence of personal perceptions, values, and beliefs).

To summarize, critical thinking in the practice of nursing:

- is goal directed and has purpose:
- is used to make inferences and judgments based on facts derived from assessments of the customer;
- is based on the application of scientific knowledge to our assessment of the customer;
- is both strategic and tactical in its application and analysis of specific customer problems.

Thinking is a skill that can be improved, if we want to improve that skill. It is also clear that nurses have always had to think critically when applying the problem solving process (or the nursing process) to specific client situations. Now the point is to acknowledge these facts, utilize them with our customers and their families, appreciate our talent, and make our practice of nursing knowledge-based and outcome oriented.

Historically, generic nursing education has been prescriptive and rigid, not allowing too much room for creativity.

SUCCESSFUL PEOPLE COLOR OUTSIDE THE LINES

As Calvin said in the comic strip Calvin & Hobbs (6-3-93): "For some reason, they'd rather teach us stuff that any fool can look up in a book." Instead of restricting the intellectual process of learning nursing to the rigidity of the 5 steps of the nursing process, we need to encourage nurses to:

- identify and then challenge assumptions of nursing care;
- challenge practices, structures, <u>and</u> actions of nursing care;
- imagine and explore alternatives of nursing care;
- reflect on what has happened as a result of nursing care, understanding that in reflecting we are enlarging our intellectual data bank for future inference and reference.

As thinking becomes the acknowledged foundation of our practice, so the ability to make decisions and clinical judgments form the answer to this question:

What is the essential healthcare service which customers need...and <u>only</u> RNs are providing ???

Thus clinical judgments are:

- the basis for treatment;
- critical to outcomes improvement and achievement;
- the essence of a nurse's accountability for his/her practice.

"You want to explain everything by the facts that are known to you. But the facts that are not known to you — what do they say?"

Joseph Joubert, Scientist

Potentializing the power of nursing in an integrated healthcare delivery system will be dependent on nurses using an organized, disciplined, and self-directed mode of thinking. And this thinking capacity must be accompanied by a willingness to continually sharpen thinking skills by:

- examining relationships between facts, i.e. assessments;
- making predictions about what will happen next;
- making inferences based on prior experience or on a logically reached conclusion;
- making discriminating judgments that indicate perceptive, expert practice patterns;
- applying theory to practice for the continuous advancement of nursing care;
- analyzing the data base methodically so as to determine the principles involved and the best course of action;
- synthesizing the assessment, the application, and analysis factors into a new and/or more complex thought, assessment, or principle;
- evaluating all of the above for accuracy, value, and worth in our professional practice.

Because thinking is a skill that is improved with practice, it follows that gaining expertise in making clinical decisions and judgments takes: practice - practice - practice. It is worthwhile to remember the following:

1. Experience is not what happens to you, but what you make of what happens to you.
2. Good judgment comes from experience, and experience comes from bad judgment.

In today's chaotic healthcare system, with most of the risk on the provider, and cost containment the primary focus, the pressure on nurses to prove the value of their service will not be contained. We must use our consciously improving thinking skills to promote the integrity and significance of what we offer to outcome-based practice:

- clarity of purpose;
- consistency of practice;
- openness in communication;
- accessibility to all healthcare team members;
- valued participation in decision-making.

Intake...

Processing...

Classifying...

Deciding...

Clinical Cognitive Activities

Diagnostic Judgments (Analysis)

↓

Nursing Rx Plan
(Nursing Orders)

→ **Actions***

→ **Interventions***

By Nurse
or
Delegated

In summary, professional nurses must see themselves as thinkers, critical thinkers, who add a dimension to the care of healthcare customers that no one else is providing. We need to focus on developing our ability to operationalize our intelligence each time we practice nursing. We need to improve our self-image and our self-esteem with the message: "I am a thinker; and my work is thinking." That is value-added nursing today. We <u>are</u> worth it...and our customers deserve us!

AUTOBIOGRAPHY IN FIVE SHORT CHAPTERS

by Portia Nelson

Chapter I

I walk down the street.
There is a deep hole in the sidewalk.
I pretend I don't see it.
I fall in.
I can't believe I'm in this place.
It isn't my fault.
It takes a long time to get out.

Chapter II

I walk down the same street.
There is a deep hole in the sidewalk.
I pretend I don't see it.
I fall in again.
I can't believe I'm in the same place.
But it isn't my fault.
It still takes a long time to get out.

Chapter III

I walk down the same street.
There is a deep hole in the sidewalk.
I see it there.
I fall in…it's a habit (or a tradition).
My eyes are open, I know where I am.
It is my fault.
I get out immediately.

Chapter IV

I walk down the same street.
There is a deep hole in the sidewalk.
I walk around it.

Chapter V

I walk down another street.

CHAPTER 5

GOING BEYOND CHANGE

How long the road is. But, for all the time the journey has already taken, how you have needed every second of it in order to learn what the road passes by.
Dag Hammarskjold

There can be no doubt that the very fabric of American society is in turmoil as we move through an era of incredible instability. The social dysfunctions that dominate our nation are indicative of the need to arrive at new values, and new pathways for national definition and renewal.

The turbulence in healthcare is a prime example of those instabilities — an example, that affects every member of our society:

- Reform of the healthcare system;
- Re-structuring and down-sizing of healthcare agencies;
- Managed care;
- Managed competition;
- Lack of access to healthcare delivery;
- New infectious diseases;
- Increased violence;
- Increased substance abuse;
- Technological development of information systems resulting in an information superhighway;
- Development of robotics and "smart machines" for healthcare systems.

In a period such as this, when the U.S.A. is moving from an industrial society to an information society, we need to call this time exactly what it is: a revolution! And in this revolution, the future will belong to those nurses who are willing to give up conventional notions of what a nursing program, or a nursing curriculum, or a clinical experience, or what a nurse, or what a healthcare agency has to be. We must willingly move beyond change:

"Toward the abandonment of everything."
Peter Drucker

While the world of nursing is changing, we must move our nursing culture from one of hierarchy to one of community and connectivity.

CON-NEC-TIV-I-TY (noun)

1. State of being linked
2. The sense of coherence and continuity

More importantly, we must transform our work culture to one of collaboration; and distance our work culture from adversarial relationships. All of this must be done at the same time that we learn to live with...and love...ambiguity and uncertainty. Quite an agenda!

Going beyond change will necessitate that key players in nursing value the following:

- A sense of mission;
- A vision of the future that is keen and sharp;
- A need for new challenges;
- An ability to focus on goals;
- An awareness that consensus is strength and improves practice;
- An underlying faith in one's self to stay fit, focused, and fast as the world of nursing changes.

EVERYONE A LEADER

- COMPETENCE
- CONFIDENCE
- CHOICE
- CLIMATE
- COMMUNICATION

The world of nursing is going to thrive best when nurses at the practice level are left alone to be creative, different, and even disobedient. In fact, that probably is a very good description of the empowered nurse, who can make 90% of the decisions involving customers at the point of service.

"VALUE-ADDED' MEANS:

Customer Driven

↓

Customer Loyalty

↓

Customer = Boss

Taking a lesson from Tom Peters (1994), there are five virtues to be cultivated by nurses for survival in an ever changing healthcare system:

- Being willing to put the "pedal to the metal" and do more, more, more;
- Recognizing that action is everything;
- Being willing to embrace failure;
- No tepid responses - these are exciting, challenging times;
- Being able to focus on goals in spite of mayhem.

But...a caveat:

There is no gentle way to change a long-standing system!!!

So, going beyond change, means that every nurse must see him/herself as a business person, an ultrapreneur. Why? In order to run one's own show, by cultivating these skills and characteristics:

- Cross-training;
- Flexibility;
- No whining;
- Budgeting skills;
- Continuous quality improvement in everything;
- Loving autonomy;
- Seeking and manifesting expertise in practice and problem solving.

NEW HABITS

- **Be Accountable for outcomes**
- **Add value**
- **Be a service center**
- **Manage your own morale**

Ultrapreneurs in nursing, in leadership and at the practice level, are crucial to our success. A business orientation combined with a personal philosophy will produce these ultrapreneur habits:

- Always tell the truth;
- Keep promises;
- Be fair with everyone;
- Functional trust with everyone;
- Functional respect for everyone;
- Encourage curiosity.

> "Today and the future are made up of equal parts of terrifying and liberating."
>
> Tom Peters (1994)

In order for a tradition bound, female dominated profession like nursing to respond to the challenge of going beyond change, we must answer these two specific questions:

1. How do we go about forgetting what we know and what we have always done — before we are suffocated?
2. How shall we develop a systematic plan to attack our most cherished beliefs — especially when many nurses refuse to recognize that these issues are no longer debatable?

We are all responsible for building commitment to a new future for nursing, defined by nurses, and based on service to our customers. Commitment, however, is never easy to achieve and/or to maintain. Some guidelines for building commitment are:

- Weigh your commitment and the commitment of your colleagues;
- Be willing to discuss differences in commitment openly and honestly;

- Compare your objectives to the mission and goals of the organization;
- Discuss possible action areas at team meetings and invite feedback;
- Ask for and provide required information regarding decisions and actions being taken so you are not in the dark;
- Regularly discuss changes, roles, and training needs for everyone on the team;
- Consider learning an ongoing and everlasting process.

Times like these create ferment, frustration, and fragmentation by virtue of the distress engendered by tumultuous times. All team players must recognize that:

Happiness is not the absence of conflict, but the ability to cope with it.

Wisdom is always hard-earned. We are fortunate on those rare occasions, when wisdom is given as a gift, especially if we recognize it early enough. Here are a few gold nuggets of wisdom, hard-earned and lovingly shared:

- Innovation creates opportunity — seize it;
- Quality creates demand — respond to it;
- Teamwork makes winning happen — don't forget it;
- Turnover costs money, but concern costs nothing;
- Ask questions even when you know the answers;
- Loyalty deserves rewards;
- The best plans are made by the people who must carry them out;
- Beware of polishing a molehill and ignoring the mountain;
- Nurses will support what they help to create.

A noted futurist, Jeff Goldsmith (1989) wrote this about changes in healthcare: "Technology and shifting practice patterns are transforming the contemporary hospital into the critical care hub of a dispersed network of medical and social services spread across the community and knit together by computer networks and health insurance contracts."

The formation of integrated delivery systems brings Goldsmith's prediction to fruition: community based, customer driven, linked by information systems. Nurses will be the heartbeat of these enterprises. The clinical competencies demanded of nurses will be:

- A positive mental attitude;
- A willingness to be personally involved in the development and implementation of self-managed teams;
- A willingness to collaborate with our physician colleagues, and with our colleagues in the allied health areas;
- Outcomes that are measurable for our customers;
- Change management and resistance management to assure forward movement;
- A belief in consensus decision-making whenever possible.

NURSES' FORTE:

- Caring
- Touching
- Teaching
- Coaching
- Incentivizing

For Health Promotion

THE "NEW" PROFESSIONALISM IN NURSING:

- **Careers more varied**
- **Individual initiative**
- **Your development**
- **You are in charge**

Shared vision and effective teamwork can really work magic and remove some of the misery involved in this revolution. In this atmosphere of urgency, when everyone is overworked and underpaid, we must acknowledge the difficulty of marching through the swamps of untrodden territory; and find the joy of learning to survive as nursing evolves into a new and much more rewarding profession.

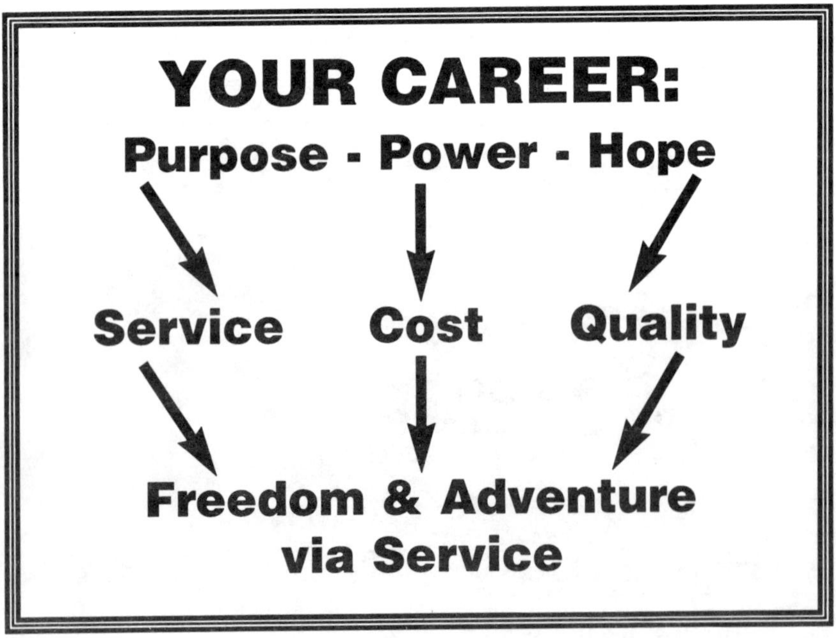

WISDOM

CONFLICT IS THE SEED OF CREATIVITY;

COMMUNICATION THE SOUL;

HONESTY AND RESPECT THE FERTILIZER.

A NORTH DAKOTA FARMER

CHAPTER 6

THE LEADER AS CATALYST

Many persons have a wrong idea of what constitutes true happiness. It is not attained through self-gratification, but through fidelity to a worthy purpose.

Helen Keller

It's no use saying we are doing our best. You have got to succeed in doing what is necessary.

Winston Churchill

The fundamental re-thinking of the healthcare industry is resulting in a phenomenal downsizing of the mid-management contingent. This change in numbers of managers/supervisors is a result of changes in "span of control," and the development of self-managed teams. Most of us worked in a time when the manager supervised 6-8 nurses....That is what used to be. Today the nurse leader's span of control has increased to 18-20 nurses; and that is projected to expand to 1 nurse leader to 75 nurses by the end of the century. This information is extrapolated from other industries, which are already heavily into downsizing, self-directed teams, and empowerment.

Here is a formula for success in the year 2002 which is based on the dramatic changes occurring in the world of work:

DELEGATE: TO DOUBLE YOUR PRODUCTIVITY

This means that 1/2 the nurses will be earning twice the money and working three times as productively as now. The buzzword for the late 1990s is "morphing" - being able to do two or more jobs safely, quickly, even gladly. The term comes from the computer industry where the transformation of images is fast and efficient.

So the "I don't float" syndrome in nursing is dead and gone. RNs will "morph" or cross-train or be multi-skilled as needs of customers, and teams, and employing agencies require. What a challenge for the leader!

NURSE LEADER'S ESSENTIALS:

1. Mastery of self
2. Empathy
3. Wholeness of purpose
4. Self-confidence
5. Authenticity & congruence

How to love the work and the job in this new world of nursing's practice - self-motivation and being able to generate self-motivating energy in the staff...that's the challenge. And in that framework, the leader is a catalyst, not a manager.

NEW CHALLENGES FOR NURSING LEADERS

- Change the name Manager to Leader
- Change the role to Executive
- Flatten the pyramid
- Consensus-Builder
- Trouble shooter
- Consultant/coordinator
- Teacher

These are very tough times for leaders: there is so much insecurity and tension along with the daily struggles to survive in a complex, competitive, unstable healthcare industry. Leah Curtin wrote in Nursing Management: that the character of the leader is most important in a time of revolution; and that the leader needs to be clear and dynamic to promote security in such a climate. She also reminds us in the same article that "giving a nurse a rationale for change is a sign of respect, not one of weakness", (Curtin, 1994). Such leadership promotes acceptance of the challenge of change by the nurse who must implement and followthrough for change to actually happen.

> People are an organization's most important asset. They should be valued, treated well, and told the truth. The employees are the ones who will bring organizations through hard times, (Curtin, 1994).

The nurse leader cannot be threatened by change, challenge, or the schizophrenic work place. The staff nurse is looking to the leader for support, for a helping hand, for a sense of humor, and for a regular reality check .

Nurse leaders need to know what nurses are doing:

- **Pay Attention**
- **Care**
- **Communicate**
- **Tips**

Here is the formula for that kind of leadership:

K x I x E x R

This formula means that the nursing leader must provide the staff nurse with:

- Knowledge
- Information
- Empowerment
- Rewards

Nurse leaders need to know when to:

- **Push**
- **Hug**
- **Cheer**
- **Boo**
- **Kick "Butt"**

Nurses at the staff level must have a knowledge-based, outcome oriented practice. They need training and retraining to keep current and expand that knowledge base. The leader must provide this support within a learning organization.

Information sharing is critical because the staff RN needs to feel that he/she is on "the inside," feeling trusted and valued, as the winds of change sweep through the organization.

REMEMBER NURSE LEADERS:

When you appeal to a nurse's highest level of thinking, you will get his / her highest level of performance!

Empowerment conveyed by the leader in deed, in philosophy, in attitude, in explicit expectation results in a staff nurse who is ready and able to make 90% of the decisions expected by customers at the point of service. As mid-managers' numbers decline, empowerment becomes the norm and is an essential ingredient of customer (internal and external) satisfaction.

The leader's ability to provide rewards to those nurses who accept the challenges of change is important, even though this is not yet common behavior among nurse leaders. There are tangible and intangible rewards and both are important to the staff nurse. The tangible rewards of money, time, and promotion are limited in a market of slow growth and downsizing. Incentives for meeting accountabilities will be highly valued in the tangible reward systems.

Nurses want most:

1. Appreciation
2. "In"
3. Help
4. Security
5 ↑ Wages
6. Discipline

The intangible rewards, like compliments, implicit and explicit power, and signs of collegial appreciation are more important than ever before because of the diminished tangible rewards.

So the new nurse leader is a different kind of leader - in all respects - from the nurse manager of the 1960s and 1970s. "Eventually, an America that had grown very fat in the management ranks ran headlong into a very lean Japan. Although it took awhile, American companies eventually learned the hard lesson: You can either be fit as the lion or you can be lunch," (Beckham, 1995).

This is as relevant to healthcare and to nursing, as it is to any industry in the United States:

- Layers of management decreased to less than six - where 12 had been common;
- span of control increased to one manager to 30 staffers (a ratio of lower than one to ten signifies "fat");
- downsizing by 25-50%;
- economies of entrepreneurship encouraged system-wide;
- move everyone remaining after downsizing closer to the customer, (Beckham, 1995).

Moving nursing from hierarchy to community within this rapidly changing healthcare system is the job of the catalyst leader:

- encourage staff nurses to make decisions at the point of service, recognizing that this used to be the province of the nurse manager;
- give staff nurses the information they need to make these decisions i.e., open book management styles;
- train, re-train, and re-train to equip the staff with an orientation of ownership in a time of job insecurity;
- find a way to reward performance and incentivize the kind of performance needed for survival in a tight marketplace.

Beckham (1995) not only writes that management is dead; but he asks why we should remain loyal to a "melting iceberg?" For this writer's purpose, the question is why waste time on a relic in nursing when the new contract between nurse leader and staff RN seeks a web of inclusion which embraces individual self-reliance and mutual accountability.

PAYOFF:

Nurses who make the money
Need to understand the #s.

Open Books

Communication
Top to Bottom

The catalyst leader's role is to move the team to a high level blend of community with enhanced personal autonomy, (Helgeson, 1995).

Thus the role of the catalyst leader is one of transformer... transforming the manager, the worker, and the workplace. Plainly said, the hierarchy under which most nurses (leaders, etc.) have developed is no longer relevant and no longer practical. If we expect RNs to behave differently - leaders and staff nurses - we will have to teach them how. They do not have the skills to do it on their own, and this is complicated by the distress and insecurity that is rampant in their current workplace.

Creating a collaborative work site, creating a learning organization, recognizing that there is no one magic bullet, and understanding that there will be moments of pure misery - these are the challenges faced by the catalyst leader.

> It is now the job to understand with intimacy the yet unimagined needs of customers and then reach out and assemble the ingredients necessary to provide them with value. In order to accomplish that, they must communicate, in clear fashion, a product or a service concept and give the organization the tools and the latitude to deliver. By listening to customers, embracing technology, and liberating information, they can ensure fluidity in a world that will shatter rigidity. It is a world that will demand much less management and much more productive imagination, (Beckham, 1995).

It will take a special kind of nurse leader, intellectually and emotionally, to not only accept, but to promote collaboration as the major force for creating nursing's new work force and workplace philosophy.

OPEN BOOK LEADERSHIP:

↓

Takes Courage

↓

Keeps the Focus

↓

Levels the Competition

Collaboration..."is a principle-based process of working together, which produces trust, integrity, and breakthrough results by building true consensus, ownership, and alignment in all aspects of the organization," (Marshall, 1995).

By focusing on collaboration and its development within every aspect of a nurse's work, the leader as catalyst will create:

- a total shift in how nurses work together;
- a new work ethic of mutual respect and valuing that creates stability in a generally unstable environment;
- a way of engaging all members of the nursing work force in the "caring" of and for customers;
- a decision-making framework that results in con sensus building based on truth and trust;
- a way of managing conflict, building ownership, and enhancing quality service, (Marshall, 1995).

The secret to successfully building a collaborative work force, is that the catalyst leader must delegate freely, give up control i.e., letting go of large amounts of power, and consider his/her biggest job to be: "getting to know his/her people and encouraging them in their work," (Helgeson, 1995). This new nursing leader values the practicing nurse in his/her new role of knowledge-worker, who has the ability to think critically, to process information quickly, and to be very creative in solving complex customer-generated problems.

PARTNERSHIP:

- ↓ **Control issues**
- ↓ **Predictability needs**
- ↑ **Ownership**
- ↑ **Accountability**

The catalyst leader builds a web of inclusion in nursing, so that each nurse in the enterprise embraces a sense of ownership that validates the work of everyone as important, that seeks to value each nurse as critical to the whole. Not an easy task in today's healthcare world where cost containment seems more important than either quality or service; and where de-jobbing is a euphemism for losing your job.

IN PARTNERSHIP CONTROL SHIFTS:

Manager → Staff Nurse
Physician → Patient
Teacher → Student
Staff RN → Team members
Leader → Colleague
etc. etc. etc.

The strategy of inclusion is <u>the</u> essential ingredient of catalyzing a new definition of the work of nurses, and therefore, the critical behavior of the nurse leader. The bureaucracy is dead, the hierarchy is dysfunctional. Long live the web of inclusion built by the leader catalyst.

> In architectural terms, the most obvious characteristics of the web are that it builds from the center out, and that this building is a never-ending process. The architect of the web works as the spider does, by ceaselessly spinning new tendrils of connection, while also continually strengthening those that already exist. The architect's tools are not force, not the ability to issue commands, but rather providing access and engaging in constant dialogue. Such an architect rec-

> ognizes that the periphery and the center are interdependent, parts of a fabric, no seam of which can be rent without tearing the whole. Balance and harmony are essential if the periphery is to hold; if only the center is strong, the edges will quickly fray. Thus the leader in a web-like structure must manifest strength by yielding, and secure his or her position by continually augmenting the influence of others, (Helgeson, 1995, pg. 13).

Yes, it is a formidable task - really more of a journey.

NURSE LEADERS:

MUST MAINTAIN THEIR BALANCE IN AN UNBALANCED WORLD:

- PERSONAL
- EMOTIONAL
- SOCIAL
- FINANCIAL
- PHYSICAL
- SPIRITUAL

The worst part is that no one - not our best mentors and not our best thinkers - has the “right” answers. But, if nursing is to have a new future, change will begin at the top with catalyst leaders who will guide our journey as we create nursing's future:

- control our own destiny;
- change before we have to;
- accept reality as it is;
- change NOW.

The nursing community must be prepared to create a vision that is inclusive rather than exclusive — and to participate fully in the tense process of change. Those for whom control continues to be both an issue of style and of substance had best update their resumes. The re-structuring organization will demand only your best, your most creative, efforts. Staff will need, and should be able to expect, that your commitment will be complete, (Truscott & Churchill, 1995).

LOYALTY

Loyalty means not
that I agree with
everything you say or
I believe you are always
right. Loyalty means that
I share a common ideal
with you and that,
regardless of minor
differences, we fight for
it, shoulder to shoulder,
confident in one another's
good faith, trust,
constancy, and affection.

KARL MENNINGER

CHAPTER 7

A NEW AGE DEMANDS NEW SKILLS

By 1982 there were approximately 32,000 robots in the United States. Today there are over 20,000,000.
Price Pritchett, 1994

You need to know that resistance to change is almost always a dead-end street. The career opportunities come when you align immediately with new organizational needs and realities. When you're light on your feet. When you show high capacity for adjustment. Organizations want people who adapt - fast - not those who resist or psychologically "unplug."
Price Pritchett, 1994

From my point of view, there is no greater stressor for staff RNs today than that of delegating the repetitive technical tasks of customer care to Unlicensed Assistive Personnel (UAP). Too many nurses do not recognize the need for delegating the non-nursing tasks to others on the healthcare team, and this has resulted in major RN discontent.

What is safe - what is legal - what is ethical regarding delegation of nursing's historical repetitive tasks?? The increase in the distress of the working nurse as a result of this ignorance is compounded by some healthcare agencies assigning UAPs to "take over" the work of the registered nurse.

RNs <u>must</u> be able to answer the question presented in Chapter 4:

> "What is the essential healthcare service which customers need and only RNs are providing?"

The Professional Nurse:

- **Well-educated**
- **Credible**
- **Experienced**
- **Well-paid**
- **Outcome Oriented**

RNs in each state must be intimately familiar with their state's Nurse Practice Act (NPA), which explicates the legal parameters of nursing practice.

The practice act defines the RN role legally and professionally. Rationally, repetitive technical tasks can and should be done by UAPs because the role of the RN must be focused on those healthcare services which <u>cannot</u> be carried out by anyone else e.g., an UAP.

The time of nursing's practice, when the RN took care of all aspects of care for a small group of customers, is gone - wiped out by: 1) the increase in RN salaries; 2) the demand to reduce healthcare costs in a reforming, overpriced system; and 3) the declining census in hospitals caused by the increase in ambulatory and home care markets.

It makes sense for the RN to delegate such tasks as those involved with hygiene and housekeeping to UAPs, preserving for his/her own practice those elements which require higher level psychomotor and cognitive skill. The customer has every right to depend on the RN to use his/her professional judgement in making decisions relative to healthcare. This fulfills nursing's very special contract with society, and preserves nursing's practice in the domains of healthcare service which are exclusively professional nursing. Additionally, and very importantly, a nurse's career satisfaction will surely be increased when his/her practice is clearly defined, legally protected, and exclusively justified.

Thus the seeds of the discontent now felt because of nursing's ambiguous distribution of tasks (a nurse is a nurse is a nurse) will be ameliorated by nurses moving into a future where delegation is just one of our high level cognitive skills.

MANAGING MANAGED CARE

C **Customer-driven**

O **Outcome-oriented**

A **Assessment & Analysis**

C **Collaboration**

H **Honesty-based**

These skills, which are requisite for managing managed care, will assist society to recognize value-added professional nursing as our special contribution to healthcare.

Putting the art of delegation into proper perspective gives nursing practice structure and additional purpose. It can decrease burnout and its concomitant problems by helping nurses to get past their fears; and learn to value themselves as the fulcrum around which caring occurs for our customers.

L E A D E R S H I P

OUR CHANCE:

- **Education of Patients & Families**
- **Analysis of Need**
- **Prevention of Disease**
- **Promotion of Health**
- **Coordination of Care**

SCARY? SCARY?

To paraphrase the words of J.C. Penney: The surest way for a professional nurse to kill himself/herself is to refuse to learn how, and when, and to whom to delegate work. Planning the care of customers along the seamless continuum of healthcare in an integrated delivery system is the major part of the RN's work. Planning means exerting control over the future, but: you cannot control the future if you are trapped by the work of the present. Nurses pay attention: we will have half the RNs, paid twice as much, for three times the productivity.

1/2 x 2 x 3

It is no longer debatable, RN's will delegate to UAPs and licensed vocational/practical nurses. And there are rules governing the art and the practice of delegation.

RN RULES FOR DELEGATOR

D **Dignity for all team members**

E **Establish a team mission & purpose**

L **Let go of responsibility & authority**

E **Empower appropriately**

G **Gathering data is everyone's job**

A **Appreciation = productivity**

T **Team building = constant**

E **Enhancing self-esteem**

Applying these rules mandates that RNs treat team members with sensitivity: treating others as we wish we had been treated.

The RN's first responsibility in delegation is to know:

- your state's NPA;
- your state's regulations on nursing practice;

- your state's guidelines for delegating to UAPs (if your state has these);
- your agency's minimum standards of safe nursing practice (ANA, 1994).

This information is first and most critical because the RN is directly accountable to the public for his/her practice. It is why we must be licensed to practice nursing: to assure the public that we have met certain minimal standards by state law and regulation.

The role of the Unlicensed Assistive Person (UAP) and the role of the vocational/practical nurse is to **assist** the RN in providing care to customers. They all share the responsibility for tasks being performed correctly. This is frightening!! Because it means that even though the RN delegates tasks, the RN can never delegate his/her accountability.

Accountability remains with the RN, as he/she assigns and delegates the care of customers to others. It also means, and this is very important, that delegation must be done within the context of the law (the Nurse Practice Act), regulation, and professional standards (ANA, 1994; Hansten & Washburn, 1994).

Today, more than ever before, nurses must learn to use their time effectively. The demands are just too great, the needs of customers too complex, the requirements of managing managed care too challenging, for RNs to take up valuable time doing that which a UAP or an LVN/LPN can do.

In order to reduce the fright factor in delegation, the RN needs to know when he/she can be reasonably sure that the UAP is safe and competent to perform assigned tasks. The RN can have reasonable confidence in a UAP, when the RN knows that the UAP has:

- the appropriate training in the performance of those repetitive technical tasks;

- had an adequate orientation to the unit to which the UAP has been assigned;
- documented competencies that provide the RN with a work profile of the UAP's performance during the training period, (ANA, 1994).

If the above three safety parameters are not available, the RN has every right, and, in fact, the responsibility to ask for these before the RN "inflicts" the UAP on an unsuspecting customer. We are talking here about the RN's contract with society to provide safe, and appropriate care, and the recognition of the fact that the RN retains ultimate accountability for this safe care.

The next safety factor to be dealt with is the RN's action when a UAP appears to be unsafe in performance of assigned tasks. When that occurs, the RN must:

- inform the appropriate persons within the institution e.g., the training department, the nursing administration department, etc.;
- document the incompetence explicitly - and in writing;
- request, in writing, additional training for the UAP;
- keep copies of the written documents associated with this incident; and follow-up so that customers are safe and the RN is secure legally and ethically.

Remember, the RN and his/her license is at risk, when the RN knowingly:

- delegates an RN task to anyone who is not an RN;
- fails to supervise a delegatee appropriately;
- delegates to a UAP (or an LVN/LPN) who lacks the training, or the knowledge, or the skill to perform the task or tasks assigned.

The RN in any state can validate the above caveats by investigating and reviewing:

- your state's Nurse Practice Act (NPA);

- your state's guidelines and regulations for delegation;
- professional nursing standards;
- legal opinion from an attorney versed in professional practice issues of nursing.

The Board of Registered Nursing (BRN) in the state of California in 1994 published guidelines for registered nurses delegating to UAPs. These guidelines explicitly conform to the legal scope of RN practice in California, which is quoted in the document and presented here:

LEGAL SCOPE OF NURSING PRACTICE

> The Nursing Practice Act defines the practice of registered nursing as "those functions, including basic healthcare, which help people cope with difficulties in daily living which are associated with their actual or potential health or illness problems or the treatment thereof which require a substantial amount of scientific knowledge or technical skill." It is the registered nurse's responsibility to use this knowledge and skill in the implementation of the nursing process: To make a comprehensive assessment (including physiological and psychosocial factors) of the nursing needs of the client, to make a nursing diagnosis, and to develop, implement and evaluate the plan of care for the client.
>
> Board of Registered Nursing, 1994

In its wisdom, and in a valued effort to be helpful to the Registered Nurse in California, the Board of Registered Nursing lists aspects of nursing directly relating to the nursing process which **cannot** be delegated, and therefore must be performed by the RN:

- comprehensive assessment;
- validation of data collected by others (UAPs, etc.);
- analysis of data (formulation of a nursing diagnosis);
- goal-setting for the plan of care;

- nursing orders and the subsequent nursing care plan;
- evaluation of the plan of care and subsequent re-assessment, (BRN, 1994).

In defining what effective clinical supervision is when discussing the role of the RN who is supervising a UAP, the California Board of Registered Nursing has said:

> The ability of the RN to assess real or potential harm to the client regarding patient care procedures is seen as integral to determining which tasks may be performed by Unlicensed Assistive Personnel. ...such effective clinical supervision must take into account patient safety, the competency of the unlicensed care giver to perform the task, the number and acuity of patients, the number and complexity of tasks, and the number of staff which the direct care RN is clinically supervising. Staffing patterns must allow the direct care RN to independently make decisions regarding assignments of tasks for a client, based upon the direct care RN's nursing judgement.

One can readily see the effort that California's Board has made to delineate the RN's role and the responsibilities of the healthcare agency in providing an environment that conforms to safe nursing practice.

The same document goes even further in enumerating the tasks a UAP **may** be assigned by an RN:

> Tasks which are judged by the direct care registered nurse to not require the professional judgement of an RN may be assigned. Such assigned tasks shall meet all the following conditions: a) be considered routine care for this patient; b) pose little potential hazard for the patient;b) involve little or no modification from one

client-care situation to another; d) be performed with a predictable outcome; e) not inherently involve ongoing assessments, interpretations, or decision-making which could not be logically separated from the procedure itself, (Board of Registered Nursing, 1994).

Examples of tasks that meet those criteria, and **may** be delegated by the RN to a UAP are:

- Clean catheterization (as opposed to sterile);
- simple dressing changes using clean technique (as opposed to sterile technique);
- suction of chronic tracheostomy using clean technique (as opposed to sterile technique).

Finally in this 1994 document, the Board of Registered Nursing in California concludes these guidelines with this very strong statement:

> ...it is the direct care registered nurse who ultimately decides the appropriateness of assignment of tasks. The registerered nurse must be knowledgeable regarding the Unlicensed Assistive Person's education and training, and must have opportunity to periodically verify the individual's ability to perform the specific tasks.

It is this author's hope that every state will follow the example set by the California Board of Registered Nursing and provide RNs with a strong and inclusive document such as the one described above. Only then can RNs really feel the security they deserve in this time of re-structuring, re-engineering, and redesign when delegation is demanded to reduce costs, while maintaining excellent service and quality in the delivery of safe, legal, ethical, and moral care to our customers.

Thus, RNs must learn to delegate: to build the nursing team; to free up their time; to increase their productivity;

...and to make a profit in a managed care system. But, the RN has the ultimate responsibility of safe nursing practice, and therefore he/she must be entirely confident and comfortable in knowing what the RN must **<u>not</u>** delegate:

- assessment (initial and subsequent);
- analysis (nursing diagnosis);
- goal-setting (critical paths);
- care planning;
- evaluation (judgement of the plan);
- interventions that require professional nursing judgment.

WHAT <u>NOT</u> TO DELEGATE

- **Assessment**
- **Analysis**
- **Planning**
- **Evaluation**

DO NOT DELEGATE:

Interventions requiring Professional Judgment

There must be no question of what is the domain of RN practice: first, for the security of our customer; and second, for the protection of the professional nurse's license to practice.

AMAZING RESULTS:

Delegate Right Things →

RIGHT PEOPLE!!

Remember delegation takes planning; and yes: delegating takes time.

"D" TAKES PLANNING

WHAT I DO	WHAT TO "D"
TO WHOM	PREP TIME

Taking the time to do the planning results in the right task being delegated to the right UAP.

DELEGATING PROCESS STEP BY STEP

1. **PRE-PLANNING BY LEADER**

2. **CHOOSE THE DELEGATEE**

3. **STATE: DESIRED RESULTS**

4. **TIMELINE**

5. **RESPONSIBILITY - AUTHORITY - ACCOUNTABILITY**

6. **ACCEPTANCE OF "CONTRACT"**

RNs must consider this to be a challenge and an opportunity to become more effective and efficient as we grow and develop in our professional practice (Hansten & Washburn, 1994).

ATTITUDE

The longer I live, the more I realize the impact of attitude on life. Attitude to me, is more important than facts.

It is more important than the past, than education, than money, than circumstances, than failures, than successes, than what other people think or say or do. It is more important than appearance, giftdeness, or skill. It will make or break a company...a church...a home.

The remarkable thing is we have choice every day regarding the attitude we will embrace for that day. We cannot change our past. . . we cannot change the fact that people will act in a certain way. We cannot change the inevitable. The only thing we can do is play on the one string we have, and that is our attitude. . .

I am convinced that life is 10% what happens to me and 90% how I react to it. And so it is with you...we are in charge of our attitudes.

– Charles Swindoll –

CHAPTER 8

NEW SKILL: FOCUS ON TEAM BUILDING

We need to get the right people - doing the right thing - using the right resources.

Connie Curran, Ed.D., R.N.

We cannot use yesterday's answers to deal with tomorrow's problems.

Charles Handy

When I look into the future, it's so bright it burns my eyes.

Oprah Winfrey

The rules, the games, and the players are new and different. We have to find new ways to deal with old problems.

Regina Phillips

Depression among nurses, who are working in this rapidly changing healthcare environment, is due to:

- hopelessness;
- helplessness;
- powerlessness.

Attempts are being made to build new healthcare organizations by transforming the nursing workplace and the way nurses work. In the American society, as well as in nursing, the development of collaborative work teams is the most important new structure being advocated. This is true because, collaborative work teams in nursing will:

- create a learning organization;
- flatten the hierarchy and build community on the nursing unit;
- empower nurses at the practice level to lead the work of the team (<u>not</u> manage...but lead);
- empower the team to make 90% of the decisions at

the customer's point of service;

- create a culture of high morale and customer-driven success.

Results from a positive team culture in nursing:

- **Quality service for customers**
- **Empowered staff**
- **Profit for the HC agency**

The development of and subsequent implementation of collaborative work teams in nursing (sometimes called self-managed work teams) enables RNs to work very productively with team members who are other RNs, LVNs/LPNs, and unlicensed assistive personnel.

For this endeavor to be successful, the RN team leader must focus on treating other team members with sensitivity. Sensitivity means nurses treating others as we wish we had been treated; not treating them the way we were, in fact, treated. That means giving up the restraints built in by a culture that was punitive by virtue of its heredity and environment.

Delegation and its legal and ethical parameters was discussed in a previous chapter of this book. Delegation combined with collaboration and its interpersonal relationship significance is the heart and the soul of success in team work. While the RN retains the leadership role (legally and ethically), the secret to collaboration lies in the leader openly and honestly sharing with other team members:

- functional partnership in reaching goals;
- equity e.g., every member is important and contributes significantly to the work of the team;
- every team member is accountable for his/her part of the work;
- every team member feels a sense of ownership of the team, the unit, the employing agency.

NON-TEAM VALUES

- **Loner**
- **Whiner**
- **Competitor**

"You get the behavior you tolerate."

Plato

TEAM VALUES

- **Infomate-Infomate**
- **Consensus**
- **Listening**
- **People-oriented**

As has already been stated in other parts of this book: mid-level managers in nursing are disappearing; levels of management are declining; and scope of responsibility is broadening for those managers who remain employed. At the same time, staff nurses have been made vulnerable by the improvement in their salaries over the last 10 years. We simply will not have the same number of RNs working in hospitals because of:

- the declines in in-hospital clients due to cost containment;
- the irrationality of having RNs doing repetitive technical tasks which can be performed by less costly personnel.

> Note to my RN colleagues: You don't have to like it to understand it!

The journey to collaborative work teams is dependent on the staff RN's willingness to make the journey, learn the process, change the culture, and collaborate in this transformation.

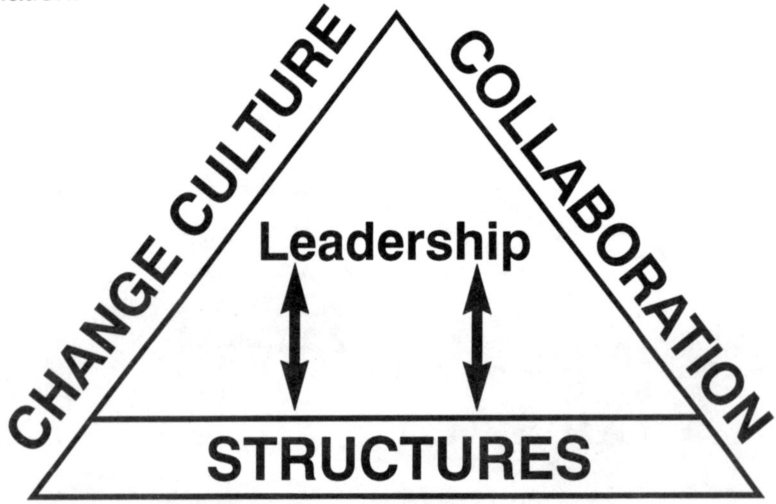

TEAM PROCESS IS A JOURNEY

The development of functioning teams takes time and great effort. The stages of growth and development on the journey are these:

- Forming: a time of "feeling out" the process; do not expect measurable accomplishments;
- Storming: a time of confusion and conflict; expect only minimal performance;
- Norming: a time when things begin to come together; expect good performance;
- Performing: a time of developing maturity toward collaborative self-functioning; expect high performance levels from the team (Ankarlo, 1992).

Why would nurses want to add the stress of changing our culture from one of "I the RN, can do it all myself...and do it better," to collaborative work teams.? Some good answers, to this very good question:

- to preserve and develop the RN work role in healthcare;
- to move into the 21st Century by redefining nursing's work;
- to emphasize the cognitive domain of nursing's work;
- to illustrate what value-added nursing care is;
- to increase customer satisfaction;
- to have the fun of innovation and the challenge of change before outside forces do it without nursing's input.

The following is a list of characteristics which can be expected of collaborative work teams in nursing:

- a cohesive, functional group of four to six employees caring for a group of customers (20-24 depending on their acuity);
- clear definition of roles for team members and shared responsibility and accountability;
- training and retraining as needed for skill performance and crosstraining as appropriate;
- shared information so all team members feel "in the loop";

- the team has authority to plan, implement, and evaluate its work based on the ongoing assess ment and analysis of the RN team leader;
- team members are involved in work scheduling; continuous quality improvement; and cost control; and where and when possible, the team is autonomous in these activities.

Working in a framework of consensus can be a highly satisfying work experience because of the high levels of trust, truth, and appreciation manifested by all team members.

As regards the 21st Century workplace, Marshall has written:

> Leadership in the new workplace must be seen, not as a job, based on power and authority, but as a function based on principles, new people skills, and the ability to engage others in coming to consensus around critical decisions and problem solving. The resulting trust and productivity will provide the enterprise a clear competitive advantage, (Marshall, 1995).

Taken at its face value, that quotation describes the kind of leader the nurse at the practice level would choose to work with. Now, the nurse at the practice level must become that kind of leader as we transform the nurse's work environment to collaborative work teams.

Collaborative Team Leaders:

Grow Your People...

Build Your Team...

Free Your Time...

Increase Profits & Productivity

The RN who is new to the work of team leading can use this checklist for self-assessment in communicating the work to be done by each team member:

DELEGATING A TASK:

(self-assessment)

Did You:

- Describe results?
- Deadline?
- Give authority?
- Clear responsibility?
- Provide resources?

A reminder from Lao Tzu: "He who has no faith in others shall find no faith in them."

The team leader must keep these reference points in mind as the members carry out assignments:

- each team member's capabilities;
- the leader's strengths and weaknesses;
- time frame for accomplishment;
- the team's check points (as determined by the team).

Here are additional reminders for the team leader, as he/she develops skill in this new role, where practice is essential to confidence:

To Be Sure

- Planning
- Flexibility
- Realistic
- Action Verb
- Measurable results
- Timeline
- Stretch
- Commitment

CAVEAT
Your job as team leader is to create an environment that lets the team do the work assigned to them...and develop themselves as a collaborative work team.

So the nurse team leader's job is vastly different from the one he/she learned in nursing school and in previous practice experiences.

TRY TO:

- Empower team members
- Encourage them
- Arrange for training
- Delegate with CQI in mind

The best team is the one that works together for the satisfaction of the customer. That happens when the team leader:

- knows the team members;
- knows their strengths and weaknesses;
- involves them in the planning for implementation of care required for each customer;
- matches the team member with the work;
- gets the team member's agreement that he/she understands the implicit "contract" of the assignment;
- monitors the work as it is done without infringing on the team member's responsibilities;
- provides constructive feedback so team members feel valued as integral parts of the team.

Can RNs rise to this level of team leadership and feel satisfaction in this role? Of course they can:

1. Nurses will rise to this challenge when nurse executives make this challenge, the challenge of the RN at the practice level;

2. When nurse executives appeal to the practice level RN's highest level of thinking, that nurse executive will get the practicing RN's highest level of performance;

3. When RNs and their teams are allowed to set their own targets (scheduling, CQI, assignments, etc.), the nurse executive can bet that the targets will be met.

Why?
Because the better nurses serve the healthcare customer, the better they protect their own careers. Collaborative work teams just make sense!

Moving to the 21st Century's mandate of self-directed work teams means diligently working at establishing these seven core values of collaboration:

- recognition and growth;
- respect for people;
- full responsibility and accountability;
- trust-based relationships;
- consensus;
- ownership and alignment;
- honor and integrity (Marshall, 1995).

Is there an RN who does not want to work in an environment that espouses such values? Surely not! These circumscribe the ideal workplace and it really will happen because it's time...and RNs can make it happen: infomate, infomate, infomate; communicate, communicate, communicate.

> **I know that you believe you understand what you think I said, but I am not sure you realize that what you heard is not what I meant.**
>
> **Anonymous**

Make no mistake, this is the future for nursing...but it is a complex and very serious endeavor. Transforming nursing's work and workplace will <u>not</u> be easy. But...it will be worth it, if we:

- simply refuse to reject this essential change process;
- deal with the stressors that will be intensified by these changes;
- handle the difficult irritating people and problems that generate resistance;
- refuse to support the status quo;
- demand the training that is essential to this new structure;

- contribute openly and honestly to the ongoing dialogue during the development and implementation of the team process;
- accept the fact that mistakes will be made;
- are fit, focused, and flexible during the journey;
- keep score as we progress;
- celebrate often enough.

THE PARABLE OF THE GEESE

Next fall, when you see geese heading south for the winter - flying along in a "V" formation - you might consider what science has discovered as to why they fly that way.

As each bird flaps its wings, it creates an updraft for the bird immediately following. By flying in a "V" formation the whole flock adds at least 71 percent greater flying range than if each bird flew on its own. Nurses who share a common direction and sense of community can get where they are going more quickly and easily because they are traveling on the thrust of one another.

When a goose falls out of formation it suddenly feels the drag and resistance of trying to go it alone - and quickly gets back into formation to take advantage of the lifting power of the bird in front.

If we have the sense of a goose, we will stay in formation with those who are headed in the same way we are. When the head goose gets tired, it rotates back in the wing and another goose flies point. It is sensible to take turns doing demanding jobs - with people or with geese flying south.

Geese honk from behind to encourage those up front to keep up the speed. What do we say when we honk from behind?

Finally - and this is important - when a goose gets sick or is wounded by gunshots and falls out of formation, two other geese fall out with the goose and follow it down to lend help and protection. They stay with the fallen goose until it is able to fly or until it dies. only then do they launch out on their own, or with another formation to catch up with their group.

My Dear Nursing Colleagues: if we have the sense of a goose, we will stand by each other like that.

Author Unknown

CHAPTER 9

THE LAWS OF NURSING'S NEW BUSINESS

Everything which succeeds, is not the production of a scheme, of rules and of regulations made beforehand, but of a mind observing and adapting itself to wants and needs.
Florence Nightingale

No system can endure that does not march. Are we walking to the future or to the present? Are we progressing or are we stereotyping? We must remember that we have scarcely crossed the threshold of uncivilized civilization in nursing: there is still so much to do. Don't let us stereotype mediocrity. We are still on the threshold of nursing.
Florence Nightingale

Privatization, monitarization, complexification...signs of the revolution in healthcare delivery. As healthcare agencies attempt to catch up with the techniques and organizational changes going on in the business world, we have to carry on as our world in hospitals and healthcare agencies is turned upside down. Healthcare and all of its dimensions always has followed way behind the business and industrial complex. Just look at how retarded hospitals and healthcare agencies are regarding the implementation of the computer industry in the information age. Just think of the duplication and redundancy of paperwork and other processes on your nursing unit.

Healthcare is the #1 industry in the United States of America. It is a cumbersome, paper oriented, inefficient system that employs more people than any other industry in our country. We have only seen the tip of the iceberg of change in healthcare reform because the information super highway, and electronic growth in healthcare via computers, robotics, etc. has only just begun. And, we are behind other industries in our dedication to our customer - and to our employees.

In this topsy turvy road to healthcare reform and healthcare cost containment, we need to be consistently in touch with "beating the competition." This means customer satisfaction via quality service...in a time of declining resources. Without customers, we are out of business. The competition is fierce. The Ritz Carlton Hotel chain allows any employee to spend up to $2,000 to fix any guest's problem (Peters, 1994). With that as a measure, can you see how far behind we are in nursing? We need to be as customer focused in healthcare as is the Ritz, or Nordstrom's or any other business.

SERVICE BY RITZ

- **Work ethic**
- **Self-esteem**
- **Persuasion**
- **Team**
- **Positivity**
- **Relationship Extension**
- **Service**
- **Empathy**
- **Caring**
- **Exactness**
- **Learner**

We need to change some of the old laws — and most importantly, we have to institute new laws in the business of nursing and healthcare delivery.

NURSING EDUCATION & SERVICE

Moves from labor intensive to knowledge-based work:

- **Assessment**
- **Analysis**
- **Planning**

SERVICE!!

The first law of nursing's new business is:

> Change, change, change. We must learn to deal with it, thrive on it. That's today's relentless refrain. But it's incorrect. Astoundingly, we must move beyond change and embrace nothing less than the literal abandonment of the conventions that brought us to this point. Eradicate "change" from your vocabulary. Substitute "abandonment" or "revolution" instead.
>
> Tom Peters, 1994

Transforming the work of nurses as well as the nursing workplace means abandoning nursing as we have known it...where we have known it. The revolution is occurring NOW. It's not debatable. It's chaotic — but it's reality. We can move out of the chaos and into the transformation if we heed this first law of nursing's new business and make it work for us. All the other laws will follow much more gracefully.

Law #2: Ignorance kills! Everyone needs all of the information! There are no secrets. Refusing to share information, out of fear or a need for power, is deprivation for both parties: leaders and receivers. The greatest barrier to nurses at the practice level becoming players and contributors to change transformation is ignorance.

IGNORANCE KILLS

- **TEAMS**
- **RELATIONSHIPS**
- **THE ORGANIZATION**

Once the commitment to "infomate-infomate-infomate" is made, it is essential to provide practicing nurses with "the score." Establish a method whereby everyone can keep score i.e., keep track of the changes and their measures of success (or failure).

KEEPING SCORE:

A Weekly Scorecard

- **Key Quality Indicators**
- **Comparisons/Benchmarks**
- **Wins & Losses on Managed Care**
- **?? Making Budget??**
- **Profit Margin**

Law #3: Always tell the truth and buy into open book management. Staff RNs need daily reminders that during this revolution there are wins and losses - and they contribute mightily to both. As Don Shula, Coach of the Miami Dolphins, once said: Success isn't final and failure isn't fatal. When we know the truth, have a goal, and keep score, we can always advance instead of retreat.

By the same token, leaders know that numbers are not leadership. An open book style of leadership means more than knowing the budget and the profit margin. Numbers can never substitute for a leader's vigilance, presence, and coaching. For example, telling the truth also means:

- focusing on standards of care...making certain that the mission of the nursing department remains one of excellence in caring for customers;
- telling the stories behind the numbers (the good and

the bad) with reference to customer satisfaction, managed care, capitation, declining success, new business ventures, etc.;
- benchmarking against local and national competition, so RNs see the truth of their efforts, or their needs to improve;
- identifying obstacles to change (animate and inanimate; tangible and intangible) and making a plan with the staff to eliminate those obstacles.

Nurse managers used to think, in the old days, that if you told the staff nurse the truth, only "bad" things could happen. Today's nurse leaders know that only when the staff nurse knows the truth can he/she help in finding answers, solving problems, creating a new workplace. No longer would a nurse leader dream of telling the RN at the practice level not to worry about the big issues (like job security, survival of the organization, etc.) - "just do your own job." Now we know that only when the leader and the environment promote honesty and openness can a collaborative workplace develop, and the team become reasonably comfortable with the constant earthquake of change.

Share the "big picture" with all of the staff. That is the essence of collaboration. No secrets!! The truth keeps all the oars going in the same direction. The big picture point of view:
- motivates everyone and promotes self-motivation for the real leaders;
- defines the winning behaviors needed to secure the future;
- promotes critical thinking in terms of perceptions, inferences, and futuring;
- empowers nurses to take control of their own career development.

However, it is only fair that finally, the nurses who make

the money for the organization understand:

- how the money is made;
- how the money is spent;
- how the budget is tracked each month (e.g., read a balance sheet);
- what everything costs;
- what the effects of change are on the bottom line;
- what the ROI (return on investment) is or how it is projected on expenditures.

PAYOFF:

Nurses who make the money Need to understand the #s.

↓

Open Books

↓

↑ Communication → Top to Bottom

After all, the nurses who make the money really should understand the numbers.

Law #4: Nurses will rise to the challenge of cost containment and quality service when the nurse leaders make it their challenge. They need the leader's perspective on the challenge, but they also need time and space to think about it themselves. They also need time for "group steering," to talk about it with each other, to generate alternative solutions, to grieve when necessary. Only then can they take ownership of the problem: <u>first</u> - buy in; <u>second</u> - involvement; <u>third</u> - commitment; <u>last</u> - ownership. And that is the key: rising to the challenge means owning the problem. So leaders have another new agenda item: make it <u>their</u> challenge and give them what it takes to make this essential transformation:

- the person doing the work must own the responsibility;

AND

- if you want them to act like it is their business...make it their business (Belasco, 1994).

The wisdom of Pogo from the comic strips tells us:

> **"The certainty of misery is better than the misery of uncertainty." Pogo**

Law #5: Change management requires resilience - on the part of all participants; and the leader is in charge of change. So leaders must remember to:

- show up and smile - your presence is powerful;
- share the credit with the people who did the work;
- know the names of the staff and call them by name: your recognition is powerful as well as important;
- follow through on issues and get back to the staff within 72 hours;
- use the phone and write notes to stay in touch and to say "Thanks".

WHY/HOW of FACE-to-FACE:

- **Use of phone**
- **Handwritten notes**
- **Give them space and power**
- **Give them time to talk together socially**

Law #6: Acknowledge that these are very tough times and share your vision of nursing's future over and over again. We all want to be treated with respect and to have self-respect. We all want to derive satisfaction from our work. We all have concerns with the way our world, our society and our profession is changing today.

The issues for all of us are:

- fear;
- powerlessness;
- self-esteem;
- security.

These issues are as real for nurse leaders as they are for nurses at the practice level. Each of us needs to have these feelings/issues acknowledged, discussed, and respected. No!! We don't have the answers and there are no quick and easy solutions. The acknowledgement is not an answer or a solution, but it is respectful and it inspires trust.

> *"How do I work? I grope."*
> *Albert Einstein*

The last law: Perception is reality. What I see - is how it is; what I feel cannot be altered by anyone but me. However, perceptions do change because of experience. Great support, learning to love the work and the job, learning to thrive in this revolution — those experiences can overcome the dismal perceptions of hopelessness and powerlessness.

The final word is from Tom Peters (1994) who says that to perceive thriving in these crazy times, we need:

- a passion for failure - so keep trying and moving in the right direction;
- a bias for action;
- a love for ambiguity and uncertainty;
- a love of the outrageous;
- an intolerance for the boring and for boredom;
- a love of humor;
- energy for the long term.

> ***To love what you do, and feel that it matters...***
> ***how could anything be more fun?***
>
> ***K. Graham, Publisher,***
> ***Washington Post***

Excellence can be attained if you:

Care

more than others think is wise...

Risk

more than others think is safe...

Dream

more than others think is practical

Expect

more than others think is possible.

Author: Unknown

CHAPTER 10

CONTROLLING OUR OWN DESTINY

No one can make you feel inferior without your consent.
Eleanor Roosevelt

We fought hard...
We gave it our best.
We did what was right...
and we made a difference.
Geraldine Ferraro

Learning and living. But they are really the same thing aren't they? There is no experience from which you can't learn some thing. ...and the purpose of life, after all, is to live it, to taste experience to the utmost, to reach out eagerly and without fear for newer and richer experience.
Eleanor Roosevelt

Nurses are going to need different skills to really control their destiny; and those skills are not currently taught in generic nursing programs. Team building skills, delegation, and negotiation skills, and vastly improved communication skills are examples of what is needed to build the staff nurse's confidence quotient.

Controlling one's own destiny means having fun, having economic security, making a difference in your work with others, recognizing that a risk quotient and a quest quotient are just as important as an intelligence quotient.

JOB SECURITY ??

DOWNSIZING

DELAYERING

NO TIME
LESS MONEY
↑ DEMANDS

It means assessing your career, your goals, your needs for professional development and getting an action plan:

Act I Assessment;
Act II Goal Setting;
Act III Implementation;
Act IV Reflection/Evaluation

DESIGNING YOUR OWN FUTURE:

ACT I → WAKE-UP

ACT II → PLANNING

ACT III → IMPLEMENT

ACT IV → EVALUATE

Looks familiar - doesn't it? As nurses we have used this process forever to our patients'/customers' advantage. Now we need to be proactive for ourselves by:

- engaging in the revolution that is changing the work of nursing;
- educating ourselves - as needed - to prepare for new roles, new challenges, new opportunities;
- reducing our anxiety and fear by raising our flexibility and fun quotient as we create the future;
- getting on the information superhighway and finding ways to use technology to make nursing's work more productive, cost-effective, and responsive to customers' needs;
- fully participating as decision makers of primary influence in this new culture;
- encouraging and supporting each other as risk takers with increased autonomy.

RN's Please Note Needed Work Attitudes & Behaviors

- ❑ **Adaptability**
- ❑ **Appreciation of Ambiguity**
- ❑ **Access Ability**
- ❑ **Accessibility**

Power is the ability to create change. That's all it is. It does not have gender; and it does not have inherent negative connotations. Power is good if the change it creates is good. The work of nurses has been altogether too focused on versatility, including all of the usual female skills of homemaking, housekeeping, and office maintenance. These historical tasks of females, combined with the repetitive technical skills of hygiene have made nurses vulnerable and kept them powerless.

Nurses are highly educated experts who are still trying to meet all the basic service needs of customers (patients and physicians). The time has come to not only control our own destiny, but to take the lead (demand the lead when necessary), in re-structuring our role.

Re-design & Re-structure & De-layer & Re-train

- The work
- The worker (partners)
- The managers (leaders)

Administrators, consultants, insurance companies are not qualified to do this - although admittedly they are, in fact, doing it. Nurses must become power players in these activities. If the paradigm of nursing's practice is changing, as it definitely is, nurses must be the architects of those changes, not just the construction workers walking the high steel beams.

OUT:

Job security & outside career controls

IN:

Opportunity & the chance to make a difference

How can nurses move quickly from feelings of powerlessness to feelings of power - in control of their future?

- PERSONALLY: Self-empowerment is the opening movement; allow yourself to feel powerful and perceive this as necessary and good;
- PROFESSIONALLY: Recognize the significant contributions nurses make to healthcare delivery; promote the nurse's expertise at every opportunity by contributing significantly and positively in every forum that involves customer service;
- POLITICALLY: Accept the fact that nurses have been remiss in the art of influence because of nursing's feminine origins; allow yourself to be a force for change via a powerful articulation of nursing's mission, vision, values, and goals.

Controlling our own destiny means willingly looking at ourselves and figuring out why we are not in control to begin with.

Ready or Not??

- ▽ **Immaturity**
- ▽ **Blame - Shifting**
- ▽ **Self - Absorption**

Whinorrhea!!

**Nurses do eat their young...
and How!**

Symptoms:

- Blaming
- Hostility
- Failure in truth-telling
- Games
- Lack of Questioning
- Fear of Procrastination

NURSES, YOUR CHOICE:

* ✳ **Cynic**
* ✳ **Bystander**
* ✳ **Victim**
* ✳ **Freedom**
* ✳ **Service**
* ✳ **Adventure**

Josefowitz (1980) makes the following distinctions between feeling powerful and feeling powerless:

<u>I feel powerless when:</u>

- I'm ignored.
- I'm on unfamiliar ground.
- I'm indecisive.
- I'm exhausted.
- I'm sitting with an interviewer.
- I'm told what to do, without a choice.
- There are too many demands on me.
- I'm being controlled or manipulated.
- I have pent up anger.

<u>I feel powerful when:</u>

- I'm energetic.
- I'm healthy.
- get positive feedback.
- I know I look good.
- I tell people I have my own secretary.
- I have clear goals.
- I'm familiar with the subject.
- I stick to decisions.
- I speak out against injustice.

- I feel isolated in a group. without guilt.
- I don't think (react) quickly.
- I have no accountability.
- I don't speak loud enough. than that of my working companions.
- I feel the height difference.
- I don't have control over my time.

- I allow myself to be selfish
- I tell a good joke.
- I'm in a supportive group.
- I know my expertise is greater
- I'm sitting behind a desk.
- I ski down Tuckerman's Ravine.

Josefowitz, 1980

The feelings articulated in the "powerless" list verify that powerlessness means someone else is controlling your future. The "powerful" list illustrates the feelings of control that enable you to be in charge of your destiny. It means a commitment to be proactive, to take the initiative. Is it scary? Yes...but worth it!! More than any other skill, nurses need tutoring and mentoring in the development of power skills.

Nurses in transition:

Making a new profession means thinking *anew* about everything we did, will do, must do.

DEALING WITH CHAOS

Much has been written about the differences in boys and girls and how social conditioning results in vastly different self-concepts. Without taking time here to review that body of literature which is abundantly and readily available elsewhere, let this summary suffice:

> For starters, men slide comfortably into hierarchical structures — after all, they were reared on them. Women, on the other hand, prefer cooperating with people rather than controlling them or being controlled by them. Men have no qualms about issuing orders or voicing complaints. Women, however, are uncomfortable with pulling rank and prefer to get their way by having every-one agree. Men handle disagreements with aplomb, oftentimes relishing the opportunity to express themselves. Women, on the other hand, typically go out of their way to avoid confrontation.
>
> Finally, men expect to be successful, and when they are, take full credit. In contrast, women hope to be successful, and when they are, often attribute it to luck or to the collaboration of others.
>
> Whose style is better? Traditionally, the male model of authority was considered superior. Macho equaled power. However, power communicators recognize that there are strengths and weaknesses associated with both styles. They also know that the real key to success lies not only in understanding the difference between the two, but in focusing on a style that encompasses the best of both worlds.
>
> Glaser & Smalley (1992)

Nurses must learn to work without a net in a time of chaos. Getting what has been called "the right stuff" (Godfrey, 1992) can be an exciting journey of self-discovery. Some of the attributes nurses must seek to attain for controlling our own destiny include:

- ease in developing honest, open relationships;
- a drive for connection or connectivity that forms

webs of inclusion rather than exclusion;

- a wholistic approach (head, heart, and hands) to work and work relationships recognizing that individual contributions are self-motivating;
- appreciation of the complexification of our society, our lives, and our work;
- recognizing that achieving a balance in life and work is essential for physical and mental health;
- valuing curiosity, imagination, joyfulness;
- valuing an ethical approach in delivering nursing in an integrated healthcare delivery system;
- Courage!!...Courage to achieve self-awareness!... Courage to know when to:
  - cheer
  - hug
  - push
  - boo
  - kick butt
  - move on

Controlling your own destiny means knowing and promoting rights and responsibilities. Freedom has inherent demands. Refusing to indulge in "victimitis" regarding the changes demanded in achieving the "right stuff" is one of freedom's demands. Giving up "whine and jeez" is tough. But taking control is instructive - being the victim is destructive.

NON-TEAM VALUES

- **Loner**
- **Whiner**
- **Competitor**

"You get the behavior you tolerate."

Plato

> "There is no one grand stroke that does it. It's a lot of little steps."
> Peter Cohen, Shearson Lehman

William James, one our country's earliest psychologists, said, "The greatest discovery of my generation is that human beings, by changing the inner attitudes of their minds, can change the outer aspects of their lives."

IN PARTNERSHIP CONTROL SHIFTS:

Manager ⟶ Staff Nurse

Physician ⟶ Patient

Teacher ⟶ Student

Staff RN ⟶ Team Members

Leader ⟶ Colleague

etc. etc. etc.

The collective question for the nursing profession is, "Can we change?" Of course, we can. And when we do change our attitudes we will change our lives and the lives of all the others we touch with our caring and our colleagueship.

> ***Knowledge is power...but enthusiasm pulls the switch!!***

Change, however, has a price. There is a price to the stress and noise of change. Nurses will have to learn to thrive in this ambiguous and uncertain period. We are not alone, the same is true for all members of the global society.

The fear and anger rampant among nurses is a direct result of the anxiety of loss of control; and the inability to do things as they have always been done. Constant re-assessment accompanied by mountains of paperwork and information overload anxiety are also prices exacted for change. We are very vulnerable because we feel vulnerable. But when we become partners with colleagues in nursing and health-care, control and power shift.

The single most important employee trait in the 21st century will be attitude.*

*** CHANGE - ADVENTURE - RISK**

Take control of your destiny. Reclaim your own motivation, your own sense of empowerment. Take time to recall why you entered nursing, and why you stayed in nursing. Those rewards are still there. They will be somewhat different - but they are innate in nursing's territory. Share your pride in what you do with nurse colleagues. Talk about the satisfactions in your work. Be willing to look at who you are, and what you do for the customer analytically. Should it be done at all? And if it should be done, who is the best person to do it, considering cost, quality, and service? This is the kind of critical thinking (analysis) that puts control of nursing's destiny in the hands of nurses.

Think, feel, and act differently about nursing because these are different times - a new age - a revolution. Be inventive and courageous and confront tough issues openly to find effective solutions. These times are anything but boring, so be proud, work hard, have fun, and retain your passion (boundless enthusiasm) for nursing by:

- seeking answers from within yourself and from without;
- having a personal vision for yourself: matching your goals to your vision and moving ahead one step at a time;
- living your personal vision by taking action: DO IT!!
- become what you want to be and do what you want to do:

  Just do it!!

PATHS TO POWER

Like any journey, the one that starts you on your path to power must begin with preparation. Good planning can make all the difference between a successful trip and a disaster. If you forget your raincoat you might get soaked; if you forget your bathing suit you might not have a good time. You need to learn some of the language and know what to expect from the natives.

On your journey you'll need to take with you:

- a helmet for the knocks;
- a cushion for the falls;
- a mop for the tears;
- earplugs for the gossip;
- good shoes for running twice a fast as the others in order to get
  to the same place at the same time;
- a hammer to nail down promises;
- a key to open closed minds;
- a hatchet to open closed doors;
- a gavel to command attention;
- a microphone so that you'll be heard;
- a box to pick up the pieces;
- and a friend for the good times and especially for the bad times.

And you might as well pack:

- a certificate of merit;
- a gold star;
- the medal of honor;
- the purple heart;
- a badge of courage;
- and a halo

for when you have arrived.

As with all travelers to new lands, you'll have doubts, anxieties, excitement, and many, many questions: Where should I go? How far? How soon? Whom will I meet? What will happen to those I leave behind? Will I return? Will I change?

Natasha Josefowitz

CHAPTER 11

PLAN B

We are at the threshold of a time in which we can no longer suvive in a state of denial. The rigid rate of social, cultural, political, and economic change in the world today has created what I call a high risk culture. In this culture our businesses and our lives are in a constant state of flux, and there is no room for safety nets. ...We must learn to work together in new ways while we find sources of stability within ourselves.

Morris Schechtman (1994)

Sadly, for many of us, long-ago dreams have become commonplace nightmares. ...In 1994 and beyond, a casual approach to continued learning will not do. ...The way you win, especially in a high wage nation like ours, is to acquire new skills constantly. More bluntly: you need to get (or stay) smarter than the next person, which means that you have to be committed, in some form, to school for life.

Tom Peters (1994)

Powerlessness is a state of mind. If you think you are powerless, you are.

Tom Peters (1994)

Motivation can only be achieved by the individual. No one can give it to you because it has to come from within. It is generated by your desires and needs, not by anyone else's. Motivations change because of life experiences and environmental changes.

This healthcare revolution which our country is engaged in provides the climate needed for nurses to motivate themselves to new mental activity for their own careers and for a re-definition of the profession itself.

How do we motivate nurses to love the business of healthcare?

Why don't RNs just get it? It's a revolution!! It'll never be the way it used to be!!!

You don't have to like it to understand it. So...Go For It!!!

Nurses have to work at discovering where they fit and where their work fits in these new venues of healthcare delivery.

Nurses (as well as everyone who works for a living) seek the following satisfactions through their work:

- an appropriate salary with minimal internal and external distressors;
- a feeling of belonging — of being on the "inside" -of being on a successful team;
- a chance to make a difference and an opportunity to grow;
- the opportunity to enjoy the work in a comfortable environment;
- enough freedom and autonomy to promote self-respect.

Ready or not — like it or not: We are in a new environment which is causing nurses to have new experiences. We need to motivate ourselves to take ownership of these new systems, and prepare ourselves to manage our careers with freedom and personal accountability.

SO:

- BE PROACTIVE
- DON'T BE AVERAGE
- CHOOSE THE HILL YOU ARE WILLING TO DIE ON
- LOVE YOUR WORK
- COMMITMENT
- PERSPECTIVE

BE TRUE TO YOU

The integrated healthcare delivery systems which will develop as a result of the tangled web of managed care and capitation requires nursing practice to:

- focus on managing customer care, rather than providing patient care;
- collaborate with physicians and all other healthcare provider colleagues to get and maintain market share;
- continuously contribute to the improvement of quality service on ever more limited resources.

The environmental turbulence in this sea of change in healthcare delivery has changed the psychological contract of employment for nurses and all other healthcare providers:

- organizations are going to be much more demanding;
- individuals will have to take control of their own work futures.

PURPOSE =

PASSION =

PERFORMANCE

GET OFF YOUR "BUT"

The RN s perception of these changes has resulted in intense feelings of anger, and depression resulting in professional burnout. As troubling as the changes have been and will continue to be, the facts indicate that the turbulence will continue indefinitely. The time has come for nurses to stop trying to debate the rightness or wrongness of what has already happened. There will be no dearth of issues over which we could argue, complain, and argue again. But arguing and complaining are fruitless, and unproductive retreats, in a time when we must advance.

How to get Nurses to move from Corporate Co-dependency to: "The future is in our hands"???

Einstein's Theory of Insanity:
Doing things the same way...and expecting different results.
Albert Einstein

When nurses take on the management of their own careers, they will make a Plan B and even a Plan C to survive as nurses in an ever changing, experimental system.

Blessed are the Flexible:
They will not be bent out of shape!

Unknown

We have to learn not just to survive, but to thrive in the turbulence. To do that, we must willingly fight the enervation precipitated by burnout.

> *Those who will, the fates will lead; those who won't...will be dragged anyway.*
>
> *Unknown*

Banishing the burnout syndrome can be accomplished by self-motivation. We must find opportunities in the re-engineering, re-structuring, down-sizing and right-sizing. This is true for nurse managers, nurse leaders, and nurses at the practice level. Staff nurses are not the only nurses feeling that they have little control over the forces of change in their work and in their workplace. Taking care of our physical and mental health will assure that there is energy for self-motivation, professional development, and a balanced life in general.

If 85% of the work that used to be done in hospitals is going to be done outside of hospitals i.e., ambulatory care and home care, then nurses must be proactive in moving their knowledge, attitudes, and skills into those domains. Becoming the managers of managed care is a great opportunity; and movement into this very broad area of nursing must be a goal for every nurse aiming to thrive in the next millennium. There will be opportunities beyond the ones that are visible at this time. Finding new opportunities as integrated healthcare delivery systems develop and expand is the key. Finding the niche that is not yet filled; working to maintain a very high level of value-added participation as new cost effective methods of delivery care are tried; evaluating effectiveness and defining quality service for customer satisfaction: that's the connection nurses must seek and find to create more choices in a fully-rounded career of multi-dimensional nursing.

> "More will be self-employed, more and more every year; many will be part time or temporary workers, sometimes because that is the way they want it, sometimes because that is all that is available."
>
> C. Handy, The Age of Unreason (1990)

The time has come for every nurse to re-think his/her nursing career. An assessment and analysis of need, might include completing these statements which have been adapted from the work of Matejka and Dunsing (1995):

REGARDING MY NURSING CAREER

1. As a nurse, I am happiest when ______________________
2. As a nurse, I love to ______________________
3. As a nurse, I feel satisfaction when ______________________
4. I would still like to accomplish ______________________
5. In the healthcare reform movement, I want to be part of ______________________
6. I am enthusiastic about the future of nursing because ______________________
7. My nursing career goals are ______________________

There are many jobs which will have no place in the near future because of the information superhighway, information technology, and data management. Some of those jobs which will disappear are: secretary; bank teller; telephone operator; receptionist; mid-level managers. However, there are jobs which will be needed that we have not even heard of as yet: interactive advertising executive; cyber librarian;

communications network technician; network technologist; new paraprofessionals. Note that all of these are knowledge-based occupations related to the information age.

Can change be constant? It absolutely can; and this is what is happening; and what will continue to happen in the workplace in general and in nursing's work and workplace specifically. As hospitals re-structure, nurses must re-tool...and plan to re-tool on a regular basis. This is a permanent condition analogous to white water rafting. Re-inventing your career is essential in nursing as your workplace continues to shake, rattle and roll on:

1. Be willing to be unusual...even daring;
2. Be fast and capitalize on the changes occurring in your workplace;
3. Be non-traditional in how you perceive your role/roles;
4. Be willing to slay some sacred cows;
5. Be aware that your mental anchors can hold you back;
6. Be willing to become a leader because management as a career is dying;
7. Be an "insider" whenever possible — be willing to do more than the average nurse, nurse manager or nurse leader;
8. Stay in school;
9. Never stop growing — seek every opportunity for personal and professional development;
10. Become computer literate as part of your lifelong learning program for success;
11. Be curious — use your imagination;
12. Find yourself a coach;
13. Find yourself a mentor;
14. Seek out <u>positive</u> people and professional colleagues - stay away from negaholics (chronic negative copers);
15. Be a willing coach and mentor to others.

Making The Most of Each Action Step
"Commitment is what transforms a promise into reality. It is the words that speak boldly of your intentions, and the actions which speak louder than the words. Commitment is the stuff character is made of."
Shearson Lehman/American Express

Being proactive in career development means being willing to set goals and make an action plan for implementation. Use this action plan to start your new explorations and movements:

ACTION PLAN			
My Needs For Improvement	My Plans For Improvement	Quarterly Follow-Up (add comments)	
		FIRST QUARTER	SECOND
1.			
2.			
3.			

It is critical that nurses work with the changes that result from re-structuring and fiscal constraints. Protecting your own career means surveying your "DATA" and recycling as necessary:

- D: Desires
- A: Abilities
- T: Temperament
- A: Assets (Bridges, 1994).

REMEMBER:

BEING AVERAGE HAS NO APPEAL TO A REAL LEADER!

Nursing's new circulatory system (as a result of the "dejobbing" that is occurring in hospitals) means looking for redeployment opportunities in the community. Opportunities like these:

- all elder services;
- all aspects of home care (pre-hospital as well as post hospital);
- community nursing clinics;
- private duty;
- infusion therapy;
- case management;
- all aspects of nursing continuing education;
- all aspects of health and wellness promotion;
- all aspects of disease prevention.

"Lifelong learning is the only way to stay competitive in the job market."

Tom Peters

Re-cycling careers in the age of de-jobbing in the information age is not unique to nurses. It means recognizing that new times and new problems require new solutions and it means re-inventing our work to conform to new demands. It is scary — but see the excitement in it too.

NURSES IN TRANSITION:

Making a new profession means thinking *anew* about everything we did, will do, must do.

DEALING WITH CHAOS

> ***The old rules are gone — but the new rules are not yet clear.***
>
> ***William Bridges***

As nurses move into community nursing practice, their job search skills need sharpening. Searching for work is new territory for nurses and adds to the stressors already discussed in this changing world of healthcare. Nurses must focus their pre-planning for job search on:

- acquiring all the information available on the area of interest;
- prioritizing that which is of greatest interest;
- doing additional research including networking with other nurses in the new venues;
- preparing a complete, professional resume that represents your professional life thus far;
- preparing for the interview (dress, questions, body

language, responses: practice; practice; practice);
- know who the power players and gatekeepers are in the areas you are investigating;
- don't be afraid to pursue i.e., gentle "nagging," to manifest your persistence and interest;
- following up every contact with a handwritten note of thanks;
- be sure you have a professionally prepared business card to leave after every visit and to place in every note;
- do your homework and always be prepared (Richardson, 1995).

> ***"Constant training, re-training, job-hopping, and even career-hopping, will become the norm."***
>
> ***Devereaux and Johansen***

Professional development means being willing to move into a new future — as yet undefined — but definitely different in all aspects from our training and basic education. Professional development means:
- a high interest in professional growth;
- adaptivity;
- durability;
- emphasizing nursing's uniqueness to customer life-time value;
- recognizing "value-added" nursing as contributing more than we cost.

Nurses who are growing and changing as they seek professional development are looking for "Plan B" career opportunities. "Plan A" was nursing as we knew it. "Plan B" is our place in the redefined nursing profession:

"PLAN B" CAREER PROGRAM"

- Accept the need for change.
  - Define your sense of purpose and your career goals.
  - Create your personal vision of the future.
  - Set and track your priorities: be action oriented.

JUST DO IT!!!

As you seek to adjust — to be flexible — to be passionate in taking charge of change, remember: all change is self change! The great danger is allowing "inner kill" to demotivate you. "Inner kill" according to Leider (1994) is:

- not growing;
- avoiding decisions;
- daydreaming about retirement;
- doing nothing, but talking, talking, talking, talking about doing something;
- talking about the same things every day.

"INNER KILL is the death of self-respect."

Richard Leider

Face the ultimate challenge by assessing your strengths and your talents and taking charge of change for yourself.

NOW: THE ULTIMATE CHALLENGE

<u>You</u> must make it happen; dreams become reality via ACTION:

1.

2.

3.

Vision without action is dreaming. Make something happen. Do not become part of nursing's working wounded. And if you are that already — give up your confusion, your anxiety, your anger...and move into a new era (Cabrera & Albrecht, 1995). Job security today is focused on value-added attitudes and value-added skills.

In summary, career management for nurses is a process focused on:

- self-assessment;
- goal setting;
- alignment of assessment with goals;
- market assessment for what is best for you;
- skill strengthening;
- action planning;
- implementation and review (Cabrera & Albrecht, 1995).

SKILL STRENGTHENING

Functional skills

Administrative skills

Personal skills

Technical skills

WHERE - WHY - HOW

IMPLEMENTATION:

- Get out & about
- Leaders are readers
- School is a tool
- Practice
- Become a "Joiner"
- Network

YOU DRIVE YOUR CAREER!! - Review!!

<u>THE PLAN</u>

- **Accept reality as it is.**
- **Change before you have to.**
- **Raise your self confidence.**
- **Choose a mentor.**
- **Volunteer.**
- **Give up denial.**
- **Get focused.**

Final words of wisdom:

1. You don't have to like it to understand it!
2. C+ just doesn't cut it today!
3. "I don't float" syndrome = inner kill!
4. Curing professional malaise in nursing is Job #1 and must be done by nurses!
5. Beware of solving the wrong problem!
6. Prepare for the race!
7. Hold yourself accountable!
8. Toughen up!
9. Face your fears!
10. Become an eagle!!!

A NURSE'S AFFIRMATION

I AM A WONDERFUL, CAPABLE, COMPETENT PERSON.

I BELIEVE IN MYSELF AND IN MY CAPABILITIES.

I BELIEVE IN NURSING AS AN OCCUPATIONAL FORCE FOR SOCIAL GOOD.

I KEEP MYSELF WELL-PREPARED IN KNOWLEDGE AND SKILLS AND I MAINTAIN AN ATTITUDE THAT ALLOWS ME TO PERFORM TO THE UTMOST OF MY ABILITY.

I BELIEVE IN NURSING AS A CAREER NOT JUST A JOB.

I BELIEVE IN MYSELF AND IN MY NURSING COLLEAGUES.

I BELIEVE THAT NURSING'S MAXIMUM CONTRIBUTION FOR SOCIAL BETTERMENT WILL BE ACHIEVED THROUGH UNITY AND MAINTAINED WITHIN OUR DIVERSITY.

I WORK TO SUPPORT MY COLLEAGUES THROUGH NETWORKING.

I BELIEVE IN OUR PROFESSIONAL ORGANIZATIONS AS A MEANS OF ACHIEVING COLLECTIVE POWER AND INFLUENCE.

I CELEBRATE EACH ACHIEVEMENT MADE BY MY NURSING COLLEAGUES, FOR EVERY HONOR FOR NURSING, HONORS ME AS WELL.

ANONYMOUS

CHAPTER 12

THE PASSWORD IS CHANGE

The real challenge is not so much to learn new things; but to unlearn old things.

Peter Senge, The Fifth Discipline

We live in a time as nurses when everything we have learned in the past about healthcare delivery is changing. Actually, the changes have already happened, and we are racing to understand them. However, many nurses are having trouble letting go of the old ways and embracing new ones. But all aspects of the healthcare system are under scrutiny; and nurses are being forced to look at their work and their jobs differently.

Hammer and Stanton in The Reengineering Revolution (1995) give these lessons on change management:

- Leadership is the primary ingredient;
- Leadership must exemplify commitment;
- Executive management must see consensus as a requirement;
- Vigilance must be constant;
- All change represents loss to participants;
- "If you believe you can't change, you won't" (Hammer & Stanton, 1995).

If the password to the future is change itself, and if leadership is the primary ingredient in a successful journey, then managing resistance is the major task of leaders. For example, leaders must help nurses keep score on successes, so that the progress of change is monitored by everyone involved in creating new roles for nurses.

KEEPING SCORE:

- Key quality indicators
- Comparisions
- Wins & Losses on Managed Care
- ?? Making budget ??
- Profit margin

Leaders must constantly remind nurses that ignorance is the greatest barrier to our growth as a profession. Therefore all practicing nurses need to know that numbers, i.e., budgets, in and of themselves are not a substitute for leadership. We must also, concentrate on the following:

- Setting and maintaining high standards for quality and service in nursing care;
- Tell the stories behind the numbers so the numbers are real and not abstract;
- Benchmark our unit's practices against our competition whenever possible;
- Identify obstacles and work to eliminate them together;
- When possible, look for profit in problems (Stack, 1994).

Reducing resistance to change is the most important issue in nursing today as we re-define our profession's function and practice. Hammer and Stanton (1995) provide these cues to leaders working to overcome resistance:

- Incentives: positive and negative;
- Information: to decrease fear, uncertainty and doubt;
- Intervention: face to face whenever possible;
- Indoctrination: keep working on the process of change as inevitable;
- Involvement: give every nurse the chance to be part of the change effort.

The art of selling the change process is the leader's greatest challenge; and it is a performing art. Performing arts require skill and presence as part of the visibility of the leader. It is the visibility of the leader as a communicator which makes the role artful.

In these days of de-layering, de-jobbing and re-structuring, nurses are raising huge barricades in maintaining resistance to change. Leaders must confront and deal with these communication challenges:

- Disbelief of the need for change;
- Fear of layoffs;
- Gossip and the rumor mill;
- Complexification;
- Catastrophyzing & awfulizing;
- Skepticism & cynicism;
- A history of poor relationships with nurse managers;
- Absence of a strong nursing culture within the organization.

Mastering the art of dealing with resistance to change only happens over time:

"When cooperation does appear, it does so suddenly and unpredictably after a long period of stasis."
Glance & Huberman in Scientific American

The leaders safety valve lies in continuing to "walk the talk" no matter what else is going on.

"WALK THE TALK"

- PATIENCE
- JOY
- EMPOWERMENT
- HONESTY
- OPENNESS
- TRUST

VISIONING

"Walking the talk" means having a serious belief in open book styles where truth-telling is an expectation.

Principles to bear in mind when communicating with the staff nurses who must carry out the changes are:

- Use as many senses as possible;
- Be very clear;
- Honesty is the only policy...so always tell the truth;
- Use emotion too, not only logic;
- Heal, console and encourage;
- Make the message tangible and meaningful at the personal level;
- Communicate maximally;
- Listen - listen - listen;
- Acknowledge feelings (Hammer & Stanton, 1995).

When these principles are utilized consistently, there will be tremendous payoffs in the form of trust and change...over time.

OPEN BOOK
"MANAGEMENT"
↓
Takes Courage
↓
Keeps the Focus
↓
Levels the Competition

"If there is no transformation inside each of us, all the structural change in the world will have no impact on our institutions." Block in Stewardship, 1993.

Organizational change in nursing and in nursing's work will mean people changes, because after all, nurses are simply people who have the same problems with resistance that all others in the American society are having right now. The service strategy in an information society will reform nursing and healthcare agencies in the very near future. Those changes will be comprised of the following factors:

- Healthcare agencies will be flattened (less bureau cracy);
- An empowerment culture for nurses at the practice level;

- Information, information, information (shared openly and often);
- Pay will be based on outcomes achieved;
- Equity will be more important than privilege;
- Customer lifetime value (Block, 1993).

These changes which must occur in nursing and in individual nurses are substantial. They will not occur automatically and will require leadership effort over the long term to be accomplished. Nurse leaders will have to help the nurse at the practice level to:

- Define required behaviors;
- See themselves as critical to success in the new healthcare agency;
- Educate and retrain as often as necessary;
- Help the practicing nurse to evaluate compliance with the new healthcare mandates.

Nurses at the practice level and leaders must see themselves in a partnership willing to grow and change in a developing system for which few have solid answers. There are no quick and easy solutions to these complexities. Block (1993) has written: "We are reluctant to let go of the belief that if I am to care for something I must control it." The truth of this statement lies in the historical management role of nurses and in the practice role of the "bedside nurse." Both of these persons in nursing must alter the regard they hold for their roles.

Nurse leaders, however, are facing a dilemma that has not been faced by nurse managers: the modern nurse leader must recognize that we are asking the practicing nurse for commitment at a time when we cannot promise the practicing nurse job security. A conundrum indeed. The modern nurse leader knows that nurses at the practice level are internal customers for the healthcare agency just as surely as healthcare consumers are external customers. But we must be careful not to call staff nurses "internal customers" if they are not going to have choices in the new organization. This means that if we want nurses to commit to a new future within the healthcare agency, they must have choices as that healthcare agency develops...even when job security is not necessarily one of those choices.

With the work of nurse managers/leaders becoming greater in scope and broader in responsibility, the practicing nurse must assume greater responsibility for what used to be called managerial tasks. In order to encourage the practicing nurse to assume these new roles the work of the new nurse leader involves these three most important dimensions:

- Balancing power at the practice level;
- Partnership;
- Empowerment factors including open book management regarding budget.

As Peter Drucker has written, "rank does not confer power... but privilege to serve, coupled with responsibility." It is crucial therefore that the new nurse leader regard change as the password and exemplify that in these leadership behaviors:

- De-glorifying management tasks;
- Ending secrecy;
- Re-distributing power at the practice level regarding professional practice issues;
- Demanding commitment to change based on freedom of choice and freedom of professional development.

PAYOFF:

Nurses who make the money
Need to understand the #s.

⇩

Open Books

⇩

Communication
Top to Bottom

When paradigms really shift so that change is the password, power shifts...and control shifts.

IN PARTNERSHIP CONTROL SHIFTS:

Manager	→	**Staff Nurse**
Physician	→	**Patient**
Teacher	→	**Student**
Staff RN	→	**Team Members**
Leader	→	**Colleague**

etc. etc. etc.

With change as the password we form partnerships in redesigning, and re-structuring, and de-layering and re-training:

- The work of nursing;
- The worker nurse (partners);
- The managers (leaders).

Over time, with these parameters transformation is possible. But true change, in a time of chaos, takes time. Remember, as Peter Block says: "Structural change, by itself, will fail." Therefore it is critical that time be allowed for absorption and structural change, but also for people change (much the harder kind of change).

Successful change within the world of nursing and healthcare agencies means:

- Structural change;
- Systemic change;
- Skills changes.

These three dimensions of change must occur in nurses and their professional and personal behaviors.

It is generally agreed that outcomes will be the definitive measurement of success in capitated systems of healthcare delivery. It must also be recognized that the behaviors of nurses at the practice level will be a distinguishing factor in the success or failure of outcomes achievement. Nurses therefore must be involved in outcomes development.

OUTCOMES

- Results defined by team
- Quantify value & quality
- Keep measures in perspective
- Share "Outcomes" widely
- Let "Outcomes" drive reform

Having the practicing nurse involved in the development of outcomes is the surest means to success in designing the new healthcare system. Because even in nursing, money is the message in capitated forms of healthcare delivery. When nurses are involved in outcomes development, i.e., when nurses are involved in stating the "numbers" that must be achieved, you can be sure their efforts will be directed toward achieving those numbers.

EVEN IN NURSING,

MONEY IS THE MESSAGE:

- **ECONOMIC LITERACY**
- **BUDGET ACCOUNTABILITY**
- **SPENDING AUTHORITY**
- **EFFECTIVE CONTROLS & MEASURES**
- **THE ABSOLUTE TRUTH**

Accepting change as the password in the development of nursing as a profession means that nurses will finally accept control of their own careers. Thus providing them and their careers with purpose - power - hope. This means: freedom, challenge, and ultimate service to our customers.

YOUR CAREER:

Purpose - Power - Hope

Service **Cost** **Quality**

Freedom & Adventure via Service

A REMINDER: YOU ARE SOMEBODY

After a while you learn the difference, the subtle difference,
Between holding a hand and chaining a soul;
And you learn that love doesn't mean leaning
And company doesn't always mean security;
And you begin to learn that kisses aren't contracts
And presents aren't promises;
And you begin to accept your defeats
With your head up and your eyes ahead,
With the grace of an adult, not the grief of a child.
And you learn to build all your roads on today
Because tomorrow's ground is too uncertain for plans,
And futures have a way of falling down in midflight.
After a while you learn that even sunshine burns
If you get too much.
So plant your own garden and decorate your own soul,
Instead of waiting for someone to bring you flowers.
And you learn that you really can endure...
That you really are strong...
And you really do have worth.

Veronica A. Shoffstall

REFERENCES

Alfaro-LeFevre, R., Critical Thinking in Nursing (Philadelphia: W.B. Saunders, 1995).

American Nurses' Association, Registered Professional Nurses and Unlicensed Assistive Personnel (Washington D.C.: ANA, 1994).

Ankarlo, L., Implementing Self-Directed Teams (Boulder: Career Track, 1992).

Beckham, J.D., "The Death of Management," Healthcare Forum Journal, July/August 1995, 38:4, 14-23.

Belasco, J. and R. Stayer, Flight of the Buffalo (NY: Warner Books, 1994).

Berger, L. and M. Sikora, The Change Management Handbook (NY: Irwin, 1995).

Board of Registered Nursing, "Unlicensed Assistive Personnel", (Sacramento, CA: 1994).

Bridges, J., Job Shift (Menlo Park, CA: Addison Wesley, 1994).

Block, P., Stewardship (S.F.: Barrett & Koehler, 1993).

Boucher, J., How To Love The Job You Hate (Nashville: Thomas Nelson, 1994).

Cabrera, J. and C. Albrecht, The Lifetime Career Manager (Holbrook, MA: Adams, 1995).

Champy, J., Reengineering Management (NY: Harper Collins, 1995).

Curtin, L., "Leadership in Tough Times," Nursing Management, 1995, 25:11, 7-8.

DeBono, E., DeBono's Thinking Course (NY: Facts on File, Inc., 1994).

Drucker, P., "The Age of Social Transformation," The Atlantic Monthly, November 1994.

Glaser, C.B., and B. Smalley, More Power to You (NY: Time Warner, 1992).

Godfrey, J., Our Wildest Dreams (NY: Harper Collins, 1992).

Goldsmith, J., "A Radical Prescription for Hospitals," Harvard Business Review, 1989; 89:3, 107.

Hammer, M. and S. Stanton, The Reengineering Revolution (NY: Harper Collins, 1995).

Handy, C., The Age of Unreason (Boston: Harvard Business Press, 1990).

Hansten, R. and M. Washburn, Clinical Delegation Skills (Maryland: Aspen, 1994).

Helgeson, S., The Web of Inclusion (NY: Doubleday, 1995).

Josefowitz, N., Paths to Power (Menlo Park, CA: Addison Wesley, 1980).

Leider, R., Life Skills (San Diego: Pfeiffer, 1994).

Long Beach Memorial Medical Center, "Strategic Planning for Carelines," Long Beach, CA: 1995.

Marshall, E., Transforming The Way We Work (NY: American Management Association, 1995).

Matejka, K. and R. Dunsing, The Millennium (NY: Amacom, 1995).

Modern Healthcare, Editorial (Chicago: Crain Publications, May 15, 1995).

Modern Healthcare, Editorial (Chicago: Crain Publications, June 12, 1995).

Morrow, L., Time Magazine, March 29, 1993.

Peters, T., Seminar (New York: Vintage, 1994).

Peters, T., The Pursuit of WOW (New York: Vintage, 1995).

Pritchett, P., New Work Habits For A Radically Changing World (Dallas: Pritchett & Associates, Inc. 1995).

Richardson, B., Job Smarts (NY: Vintage, 1995).

Schechtman, M., Working Without a Net (NY: Prentice Hall, 1994).

Stack, J., The Great Game of Business (NY: Doubleday, 1992).

Toffler, A. and H. Toffler, The Politics of the Third Wave (Atlanta: Turner Publishing, 1995).

Tracy, D., Take This Job and Love It (NY: McGraw-Hill, 1994).

Truscott, J.P. and Gail Churchill, "Improving Customer Satisfaction While Reducing Costs," Nursing Policy Forum, July/ August 1995, 1:4, 5-12.

Ulrich, B., Leadership and Management According to Florence Nightingale (Norwalk, CT: Appleton & Lange, 1992).